THE
STYLE
CHECKLIST

OTHER STYLE BOOKS BY LLOYD BOSTON

Men of Color: Fashion, History, Fundamentals (Artisan)

*Make Over Your Man: The Woman's Guide to
Dressing Any Man in Her Life* (Broadway)

Before You Put That On: 365 Daily Style Tips for Her (Atria Books)

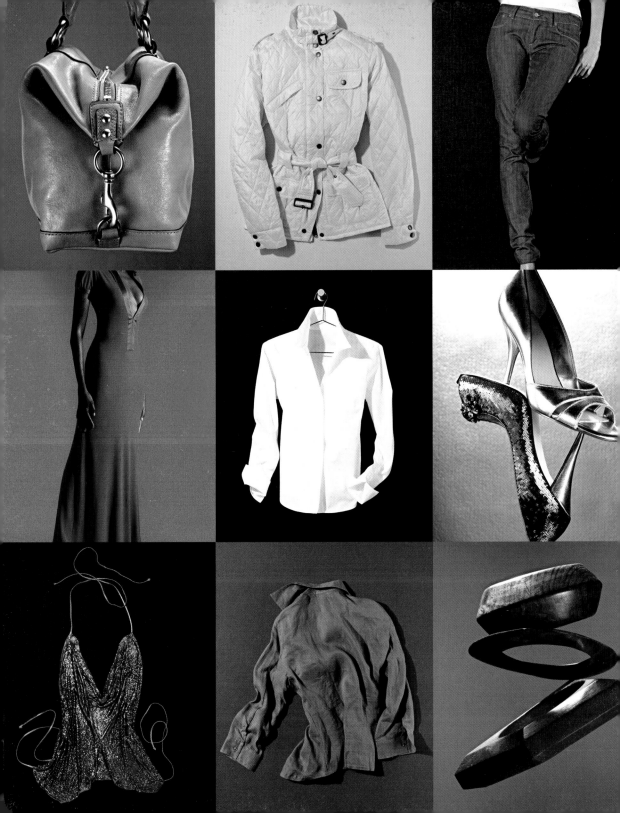

LLOYD BOSTON

—

THE STYLE CHECKLIST

—

THE ULTIMATE WARDROBE
ESSENTIALS FOR YOU

Jones New York proudly supports Lloyd Boston's *The Style Checklist*

ATRIA PAPERBACK

New York   London   Toronto   Sydney

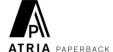
ATRIA PAPERBACK

A Division of Simon & Schuster, Inc.
1230 Avenue of the Americas
New York, NY 10020

First Atria Paperback edition September 2010

ATRIA PAPERBACK and colophon are trademarks of Simon & Schuster, Inc.

For information about special discounts for bulk purchases, please contact Simon & Schuster Special Sales at 1-866-506-1949 or business@simonandschuster.com.

The Simon & Schuster Speakers Bureau can bring authors to your live event. For more information or to book an event contact the Simon & Schuster Speakers Bureau at 1-866-248-3049 or visit our website at www.simonspeakers.com.

Art direction by Lloyd Boston and Robert Tardio
Designed by Joel Avirom and Jason Snyder

Manufactured in the United States of America

10 9 8 7 6 5 4 3 2 1

Library of Congress Cataloging-in-Publication Data
Boston, Lloyd.
    The style checklist: the ultimate wardrobe essentials for you / Lloyd Boston.
        p. cm.
    Includes bibliographical references and index.
1. Clothing and dress. 2. Fashion. I. Title.
    TT507.B632 2010
    646.4'04—dc22   2010006280

ISBN 978-1-4391-6072-5
ISBN 978-1-4391-6394-8 (ebook)

DEDICATION

To my *own* checklist of a few of the most beautiful, smart, and stylish women in my world, who have helped to shape my life and career. You have inspired and helped me in so many ways. This book is for you.

Joy Behar	Jean Johnson	Sharon Pendana
Kim Bondy	Mary Johnson	Amy Rapawy
Lynell Boston-Kollar	Wendy Johnson	Tracy Reese
Diahann Carroll	Star Jones	Stephanie Scott
Julia Chance	Erica Kennedy	Tara Simone
Faith Childs	Hoda Kotb	Jakki Taylor-Richardson
Ann Curry	Patti LaBelle	Susan Taylor
Pat Darden	Stacy Lastrina	Diane Toledo
Pat Durkin	Clarise Lee	Meredith Vieira
Rainy Farrell	JoAnn Lee	Cynde Watson
Alice Flynn	Katie Maloney	Constance White
Dana Goodman	Evelyn Meeks	Wendy Williams
Elisabeth Hasselbeck	Lolita Mitchell	Oprah Winfrey
Janice Huff	Natalie Morales	Andrea Wishom
Jacqueline Johnson	Soledad O'Brien	Alicia Ybarbo

CONTENTS

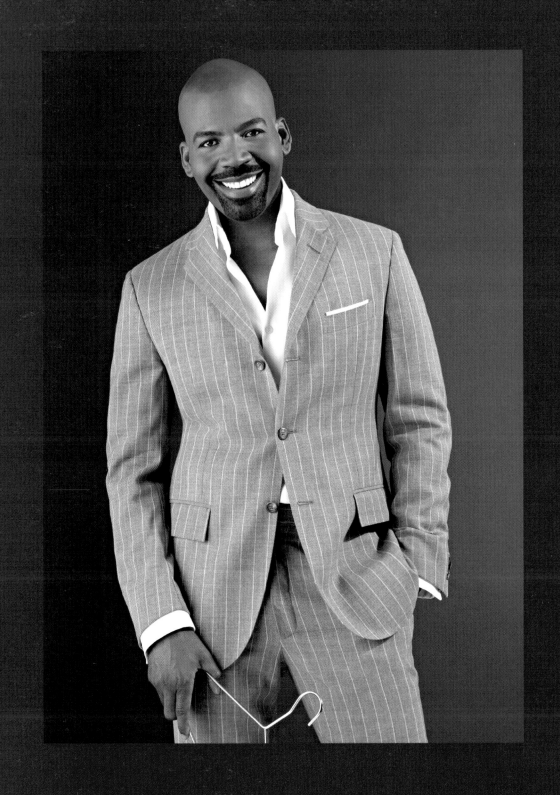

AUTHOR'S NOTE

Most women don't run out of clothes, they simply run out of outfit *ideas* and are maybe missing just a few accessories or items that the most fashionable women—celebrities and others who can afford to hire a stylist—always seem to have. I've created *The Style Checklist: The Ultimate Wardrobe Essentials for You* to unlock the secrets to great personal styling for any woman who desires to look her best—not just those with wealth and access to fashion insiders like myself.

I like to think of this book as a *prequel* to my last popular style book, *Before You Put That On: 365 Daily Style Tips for Her*. I had assumed when writing that book that most readers already owned the items that comprised the outfit combinations that I prescribed each day. In the five years since its publication, I realized that my assumption was wrong. So, with this book I'm now taking a few stylish steps back in order to help you to take a fashion step forward.

Many of us believe that the more clothing you have, the better off you are. But notably stylish women can attest to the exact opposite. Global fashion icon and editor in chief of American *Vogue* magazine (and assumed clotheshorse) Anna Wintour agrees. "I get a few key pieces each season and wear them a lot."

Wintour goes on to say that "the amazing golden years that everyone in the industry was enjoying were fantastic from a business point of view but also maybe a little unseemly. Every celebrity thought she could be a designer, and how many handbags? How many shoes? How much of a thing does everyone really need?" She's right on the money with these questions. Beyond fashion, the idea of having no more than you really need applies to all aspects of our lives when resources—be they financial or natural—become less and less plentiful. Buying more because you can is last century. Less is modern.

A myriad of choices stuffed in your closet has the potential to discourage you from being creative with what you have and make you hungry for more.

After nearly twenty years of working in and around New York's fashion industry, it hit me one day that the world's most stylish women are all basically wearing some variation of the same exact clothing and accessory ideas. Not precisely the exact items, but for timelessly fashionable women, many of the silhouettes, fabric choices, and design concepts have all been similar for decades.

I also realized that I could never expect average women to look more stylish and wear well-orchestrated ensembles when they don't even first know what pieces are the most classic. Sadly, experts like myself witness women stabbing in the dark when shopping, hoping to spear a fashionable item—and sometimes wounding their own image in the process—whereas notably fashionable women will agree that it has never been about the look or where you bought it, but about the pieces that comprise the look.

Having incredible access over the years to the exclusive front rows, backstages, and runways of New York Fashion Week, and to the red carpets of Hollywood's Oscars, Golden Globes, and Emmys, has afforded me the unique opportunity to translate high style for regular people in an accessible way. I've discovered that while women may *recognize* classic items, they don't always know exactly which ones work best for their body and lifestyle, or how to select the best of certain classics. For instance, some will choose a little black dress with gold-button detailing and sheer sleeves over a sleeveless sheath version in a matte fabric—opting not to appear too "plain." But unless she already has a simple, clean, or "plain" version already in her closet, she is making the wrong choice.

There are hundreds of these, what I call "closet classics," including outerwear, shoes, accessories, classic color combination ideas, makeup accents, dresses, eveningwear separates, and beyond. They are the most recognizable icons of universal style. And when thinking back to female clients who have hired me to revamp their entire closet, the first thing I always do is open that door and look to see if she owns a short list of certain items: from the time-honored trench in a neutral or bold color and bleach-white button-down blouse to a perfectly matched flesh-toned slingback or an A-line skirt in a gray wool gabardine—just for starters. And although the designer, cost, and fit may vary, the most stylish ideas transcend boundaries of age, race, body type, and lifestyle. Defining your style *starts* with first truly focusing your wardrobe and the place where you store it as well.

Interior designer and TV closet expert Carey Evans has observed that: "Closets started out as the reach-in design, but then the depth grew and transformed into walk-in closets" as we became more and more a consumer culture. A walk-in closet is great, but having one doesn't mean we have to fill it to the brim.

One of the best ways to get smart about style is to weed out clothes that don't fit. So many women are consumed with the clothing they have that no longer fits (and the idea of how to force it to fit again). In the process, they are missing scores of classic options and combinations that can flatter them—as they are, right now. Comfort is critical to appearing stylish because being beautiful is about feeling beautiful. I want to help you to identify the style that makes you feel *your* most beautiful, and then show you how to achieve it with ease—every day.

When mastered, I believe that style can equal power. We all form opinions about each other based on appearance; it's human nature. The idea is to exercise full control to create and present the you you *hope* to be each day upon leaving your door.

We've all done it. The day we wanted to appear "smart," maybe we chose what we knew to be "scholarly" clothes—like a jauntily tailored pin-striped suit. For the trip that was meant to add spark to a listless romance, we boarded the plane in an ensemble that made our partner anticipate a lovers' holiday. And who hasn't selected just the right top and hairstyle for a big first date? You know the top. It says that you're a catch while also implying that you enjoy a respectfully sexy chase.

In this book, you will finally have access to my fail-safe list, the elements of style and styling advice. Working with basics like a crisp white dress shirt and the perfect pair of black trousers for business, worry-free weekend warriors like a zip-front tracksuit in timeless stretch cotton, or the classic, comfortable ballet flat in a fun color, *The Style Checklist* explores every aspect of a modern woman's clothing needs. Whether you're an executive who travels, a new mom with a transitioning body, or a recent grad heading into interviews, keep this book at your side, in your tote, or near your computer for online shopping, so you can be armed with exactly what to invest in, why to buy it, and how to don it believably. The ultimate goal: Once you invest in each item from the book, whenever that is, and whatever amount you can afford to spend, you can curtail your overspending and cut back on emotional shopping by leaps and bounds.

The book also includes fun touches of history and how-tos, select celebrity nods, as well as quick outfit solutions and iconic still-life photographic portraiture worthy of framing, created by the masterful lensman Robert Tardio. The passages are easy meditations on one single theme. No skinny models wearing all the items, no exotic locations to enhance the mood, just the iconic essential, artfully styled in a photographic tribute. I want you to really feel, as I do each time I discover a great classic, the breadth of its staying power, the beauty of its design, and the genius of its form and function today—and always.

HOW TO USE THIS BOOK

Think of this book as your cheat sheet toward style. Start reading from the top, or crack it open to the section that speaks to you first—you can't go wrong. Get to know each item on the list and compare it against what you have in your closet. Do you own it? Do you need to add it? Might you need to update yours? Or if you already have it, consider it a good running start.

Pay attention to its "perfect partners," other items in the book that can be used to create easy combinations. These pairings are not the only style equations either. Use them as a head start toward countless other ensemble ideas. The more you experiment, the more confident, individual, and stylish your overall look will become. Honing your style is an evolution. This book is simply the spark and road map.

Most importantly, have fun reading and referencing it. These passages are written as if I was shopping at your side in a big, beautiful department store, really. As you read, picture us going aisle by aisle, section by section, item by item—with me teaching you exactly *what* you need and *why* you need it. The voice is my own, and the classics will now become yours!

THE
STYLE
CHECKLIST

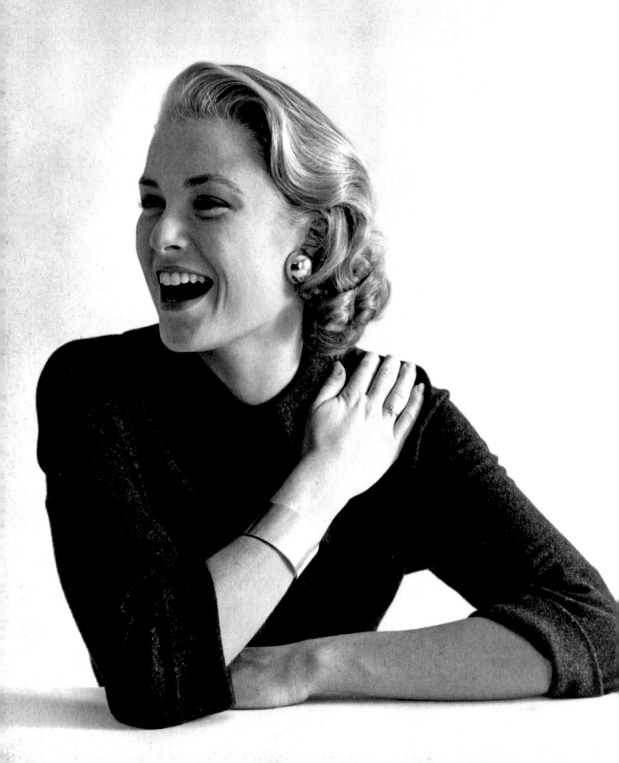

Grace Kelly

1 | WORK

The white shirt may very well be the best fashion leveling device ever. This simple neutral welcomes a pairing with just about any color or pattern, making an outfit refreshingly clean to the eye of onlookers.

While most women instinctually run to their black garments for any evening affair, it is the one woman who goes off script and chooses a white blouse who gets noticed. Not blaringly so, as if she's wearing head-to-toe sequins, but in a pleasing way because she cleanses the visual palette of a dark room. She stands as a style sorbet, if you will, amid a sea of dark colors, textures, and embellishments.

THE WHITE SHIRT

Many think of white as a subliminal representation of purity and light—like a deep inhale of fresh spring air.

A quintessential icon of style, the white shirt takes on many faces, from the crisp button-down with French cuffs that welcome artful cuff links that sparkle, to loose, organic kimono-inspired styles that effortlessly shroud to flatter and forgive. There are virtually no rules or limits, save keeping them as bright as they were upon purchase. So whether crisp bright white, slightly off-white, or classic eggshell, the goal is to keep them true to their original color by dry-cleaning or hand-washing with care. If you choose to hand-wash, with cotton especially, the best combination is a few gallons of warm water with one-quarter of a cup of liquid bleach and a small amount of dry detergent—both fully dissolved. Finish with a double rinse, first hot, then cold, which will provide a thorough cleaning.

Perfect Partners

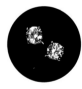

page 18   page 48   page 214   page 104   page 202

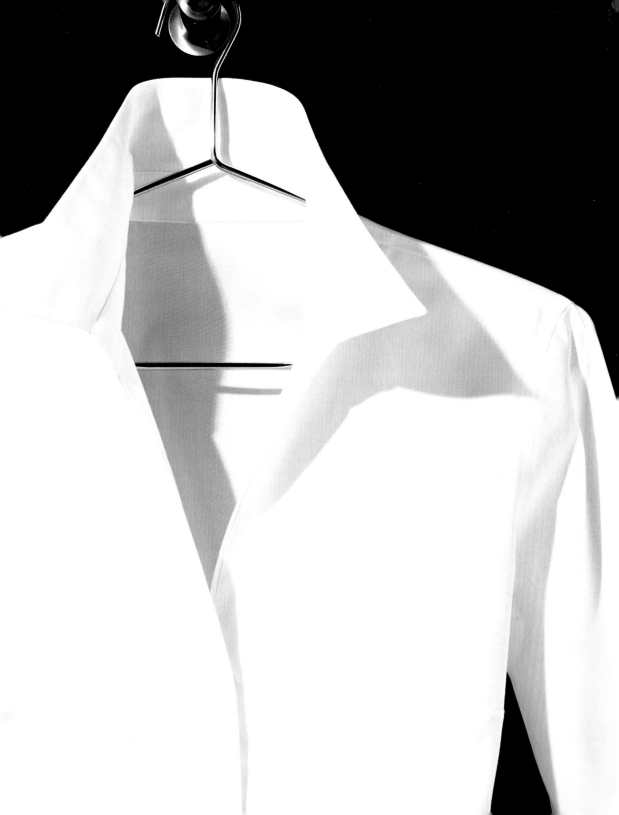

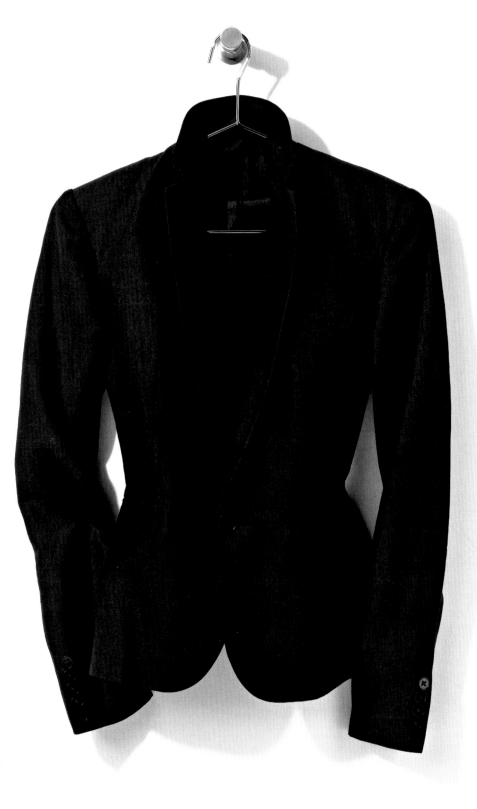

Call it prep school. Call it nautical. Call it security guard, even. The navy blue blazer stands alone as an icon of classic American style—both for her *and* him. Its stately shape, strong color, and visual messaging speak to instant acceptability for almost any room you enter the world over.

Where some may find this message stuffy, others realize it can be style power that is harnessed to your individual liking. For instance, one woman may choose to

THE NAVY BLUE BLAZER

wear her classic navy blue blazer traditionally, paired with her best tan trousers, a silky white blouse, black patent leather pumps, and a strand of milky pearls, whereas another woman will create a look that thumbs its nose at convention while using the instant-recognition factor of the jacket in a slightly coded manner. She'll wear it like a careless-*looking*, last-minute addition to her denim skirt/lace top combination. Maybe she'll add a metallic belt on top of it all, scrunch up the sleeves, pop the collar, and complete the look with biker boots and navy opaque tights. She's the girl who may have gotten expelled from prep school but still knows the power of all of its wares and pillars.

When you add a navy blue blazer to your wardrobe, there are two things to keep in mind.

NAVY ENCOURAGES BREAKUPS Your navy blazer could very well be half of a navy blue suit you already own. Don't be afraid to break up a suit, using the jacket as a stand-alone. Jackets with few details always pass for blazers with ease. Look for a single-button closure for more of a chance to effectively take it from casual to elegant. A slightly shorter length, single or double vents, and monochromatic buttons make it appear more independent. These attributes make for a more generic garment that can slip in and out of coupled or single ensembles.

NAVY ISN'T FOND OF GOLD Unless you are heading to a cocktail sip on a yacht, gold buttons on your navy blazer may make you look more like Mr. Howell—as in the character on *Gilligan's Island*—than you would like. Gilded hardware on your jacket can be a fun, tongue-in-cheek take on classic nautical-meets-preppy style, but be careful, for its potentially costumey overtones can add years to your look. This choice can also rob you of the many modern possibilities that a simpler version of the jacket welcomes. This is one instance where gold isn't necessarily golden. Start with matching buttons first.

Sweet, sophisticated, iconically American, and conservative, the classic twinset may fool you into thinking that it's a relic of the past. It is a signature garment of the 1950s "sweater girl"—you know, the girl who never revealed too much but always let you know what she had to offer through a snugly fitted silhouette.

THE TWINSET

The best twinsets are versatile enough to allow the wearer to separate them in an instant or conjoin them as designed without hesitation. The outer layer is usually referred to as a cardigan, for its traditional button-front design, whereas the underlayer can be anything from a cap-sleeve T-shirt silhouette to a tank top.

Dressier versions in cashmere are style staples that can take you from sporty days, topping off shapely dark denim, to chic evenings when worn monochromatically atop a silk taffeta ball-gown skirt. Both of these looks say luxe without appearing like you tried too hard.

Twinsets are seasonless and versatile and can benefit from strong embellishments, such as bugle beading, sequins, embroidered details, and artful buttons—the list goes on and on. But be forewarned: *Busy details may add years to your look* unless you make a conscious effort to either break up more ornate twinsets or add youth to your choice of bottom—for example, sexy dark jeans or stretch satin pants.

This is not to say that all embellished twinsets are old-lady-like. But make sure that you invest in a basic sweater set first, then add more creative versions if you choose. This is how you shop smart and build a great wardrobe. Break the embellished set to use the cardigan as a jacket replacement, and use the tank or T-shirt—a cool alternative to a stuffy blouse—beneath your more tailored suits.

And like most real twins, they usually hate to be mistaken for each other, so to get the most style mileage, look for "fraternal" twinsets, where each piece has its own distinct attributes. The cardigan may be slightly longer; its partner may have a grosgrain ribbon trim at the neck. This will give you the ability to see them as both separates and a dynamic wardrobe duo.

Perfect Partners

page 9   page 103   page 107   page 157   page 218

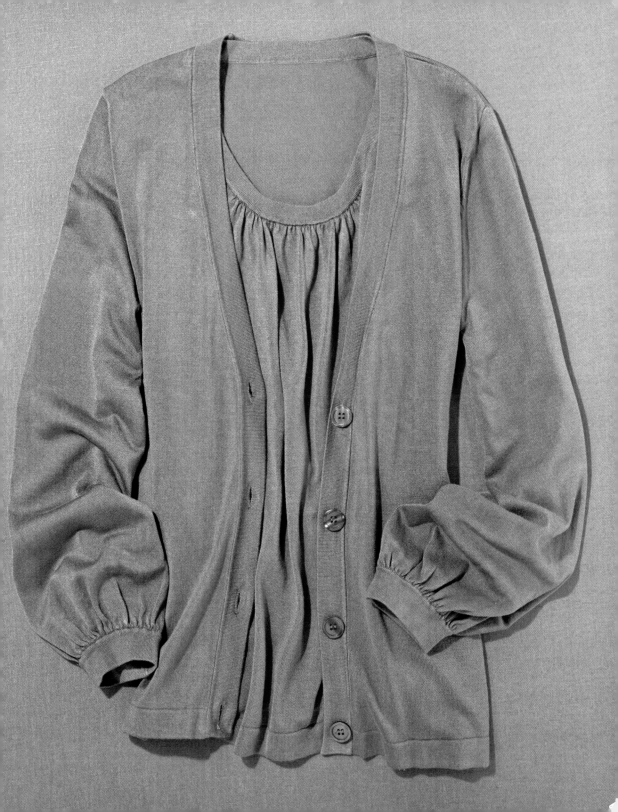

The black skirt not only is a benchmark of tasteful, tailored dressing and timeless elegance, it is also one of the key ingredients of a successful business style—ever appropriate.

What makes it register as a style icon that "grows you up" is the simple fact that the black skirt isn't always the instinctive choice of younger women, who more often opt for

THE BLACK SKIRT

something colorful, sweet, and frilly. But when you have turned that proverbial corner in life, going from "new girl in town" to "woman destined to run this town," the black skirt can go with you. Sweet can only get you but so far.

The perfect black skirt for you is the one that hugs your lower half just right. The fit on your hips is the first and most important factor.

In cooler months, this skirt calls for matching black opaque tights and black patent pumps that make other girls swoon in silence. Choose a year-round-weight fabric, such as wool gabardine, and combine it with a pale or pastel, tissuelike top and flesh-toned shoes to keep it breezy in warm weather. Here are some pointers for choosing the best silhouette for you.

BODY TYPE	STYLE	BENEFIT(S)
bold shoulders	pleated, A-line, circle	accentuates hips, balances shoulders
slim, pear shaped	trumpet, wrap, soft A-line	balances hips
boyish, straight	pleated, A-line, mini, wrap	adds curves to lower half
hourglass	pencil, A-line	punctuates your curves

Perfect Partners

page 144   page 169   page 3   page 214   page 217

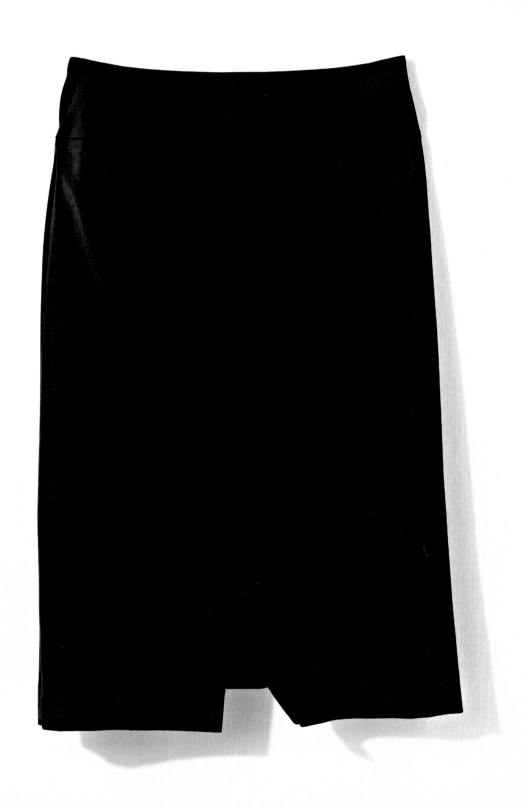

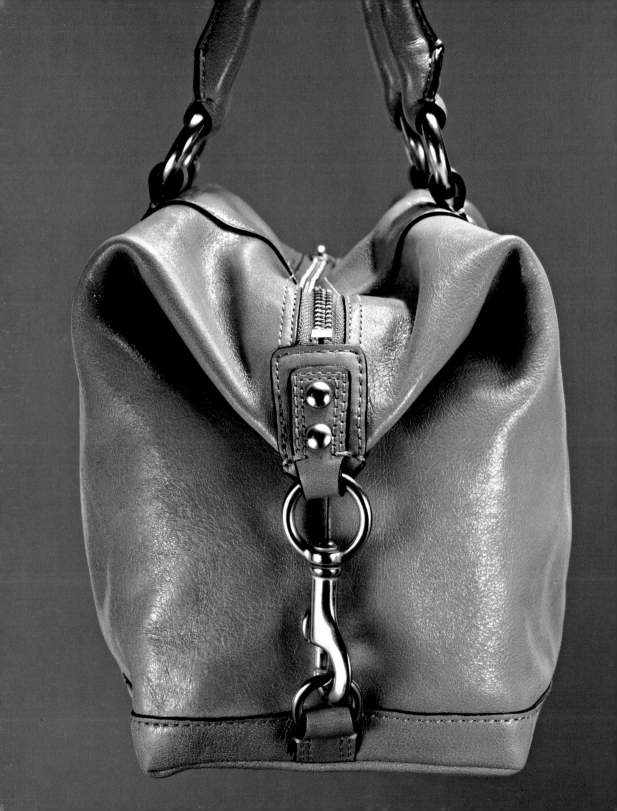

nvest in the best bag that you can afford. The return on your investment will be worth it because your handbag says a lot about you, whether it's hanging from your shoulder or elbow, or resting on top of a table or on the back of your chair.

By selecting a strong, quality handbag, you will announce to the world, "I have arrived"—as opposed to "Can you help me get to where I am going?" So choose hand-stitched leather or top-quality suede, in eye-popping colors and without brazen designer logos.

THE BUSINESS HANDBAG

If you choose an exotic skin, like ostrich, it doesn't matter whether it's real or faux. Everyone has become more green and sensitive to the treatment of animals, including the designers and manufacturers who are producing higher-quality and better-looking products from synthetic materials.

Even if your clothing is of a slightly lesser quality, your handbag can elevate your image, adding shine and value to your overall look.

"WORKING IT" AT WORK A woman's work ethic is often assessed by her choice of handbag, especially for business. The organized executive knows how to get the most out of one bag versus carrying a jumble of several bags. If you must carry more than one, stash the others (laptop bag, gym tote, etc.) whenever headed to group meetings. The bag that remains should convey the message of complete control, a touch of aspiration, and as little wear and tear as possible. In doing so you transmit a hint of your professional skill sets—even before you have a chance to display them.

Perfect Partners

page 69

page 41

page 73

page 59

page 92

Sharp. Mysterious. Beyond timeless. His. Hers. Yours. The black pantsuit stands alone confidently as a beacon of stealth style, making the wearer ready for any occasion. The smart, stylish woman wears it complete or as separates with the same security and self-assurance. This makes her modern and gives her limitless style returns.

THE BLACK PANTSUIT

Invest as much as you can and ask a tailor to fit the jacket and pants to within an inch of your life—while allowing you a little room for the gaining and losing of a few pounds.

Choose a fabric like a year-round tropical-weight wool or wool gabardine. A single-button closure will look the smartest, taking you from casual and business straight into any last-minute evening event where a dress feels like too much.

And like we've seen with every single-name style icon, from Halle and Oprah to Cher and Angelina, who's dipped herself in a black pantsuit, it knows no age or body type—when you know how to rock it right. Here's exactly how at any age.

TWENTYSOMETHING Choose a slimmer cut and a slightly cropped jacket, and instruct a tailor to add two-inch cuffs to the pants and replace cheaper buttons with top-quality horn buttons. You should also remove all the inside pockets for a smoother line. You will look like you spent a fortune.

THIRTYSOMETHING Wear it to work with flouncy tops, to play against its "mensy" tailoring. Or just feature the lean, sharp pants with your favorite denim jacket, a colorful tank, and an exotic-skin clutch for wine tastings where Mr. Right might be sipping next to you.

FORTYSOMETHING Break it up! The jacket can make your dark denim ready for dinner—just by adding a sleeveless black turtleneck, frisky clutch bag, and lip gloss. The pants can do double duty if you add your highest heels and a shimmy of a metallic top to the mix as you head for any city's hippest new lounge.

FIFTYSOMETHING AND BEYOND Choose a white ruffled top and snakeskin heels with your black suit for, let's say, volunteering at a fund-raiser. Heading to the theater? Put on a silky, sleeveless camisole—for that barely there look—then spice it up with a chunky necklace. Now, that'll give new meaning to the term "hot flash"!

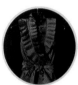

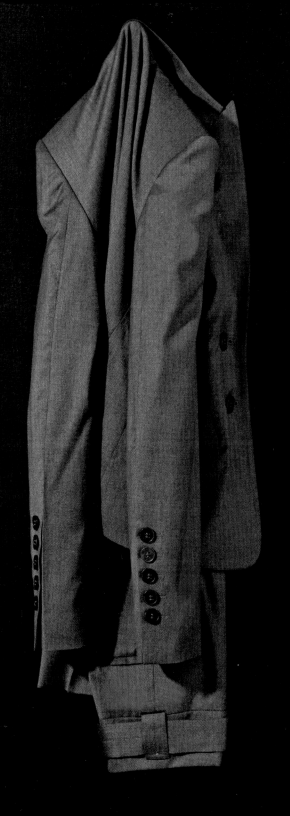

One hundred percent wool flannel is a loosely woven fabric with a napped surface, traditionally used to conceal the weave. Historically, suits created in this classic material were mainly men's pantsuits. But those days have long been over.

The gray flannel pantsuit is a great style statement for both men *and* women. You can play it casual and sporty with a flat black sandal, petal pink T-shirt, and a canvas tote. Or make it perfect for a nighttime event with a black satin ankle-

THE GRAY FLANNEL SUIT

strap stiletto and a satin ruffled blouse, finished off by a bold red lip, chandelier earrings, and a sparkly minaudière clutch bag.

The most important factor is the fit. This comes before worrying about the designer or price. Look for the following.

SHOULDER FIT The jacket should rest squarely on your natural shoulders and not grip them. Any excess fabric or padding hanging off the edge of your body is a sign of a poor fit.

PANT LENGTH When wearing heels, the hem should fall just between the top and middle of your most common heel height. If it is in your budget, invest in a second pair of trousers to be worn solely with flats.

BUTTON CLOSURES Although two- and three-button suits are totally acceptable and timeless, opt for a single-button model. The solo closure easily passes for an elegant evening suit while still working as a sporty blazer if you choose to divorce the set. A two-button model is the next-best choice.

From Minnie Mouse (formerly known as "Minerva") and her clunky 1920s-inspired versions, to Oprah Winfrey's modern-day slim, chic, red-bottomed Christian Louboutins rocked each afternoon on our TV screens, the pump, especially in black, may be the most definitive style punctuation in a well-dressed woman's ensemble.

THE BLACK PUMP

Contrasting heels, mesh sides, zippered toes—you name it, and it has probably been done or is about to be introduced. As a result of decades of redesign and inspired permutations, the black pump lives today as its own master accessory choice, allowing women the power to build an entire look around its mere presence.

For instance, a look featuring a black pencil or A-line skirt and a black pump will take on a new level of chic with the help of a bold, textured black tight or fishnet stocking in cooler months. And most stylists know that glossy black patent pumps almost scream out to be paired with your clothes in matte fabrics (not the shiny fabrics as you might assume).

There are some days where your black pumps will not only seal the deal but *are* the deal. Potentially soggy days when black or tan raincoats fill the sidewalks of busy city streets give a center-stage spotlight to your pumps. Complement them with a wide (or slim) matching black belt atop your tan trench, or by donning a pair of opaque tights in saturated crimson, Dijon, or amethyst to create a vertical visual thrust right down to your tootsies when rocking your black trench.

So, take your cue from the heel up and choose your black pumps wisely, invest the most you can afford, and never allow them to just exist on your foot. For when you step into a fabulous black pump, you are stepping into a very fashionable legacy of well-heeled women of style. Make your footprint count.

Perfect Partners

page 70   page 187   page 143   page 166   page 201

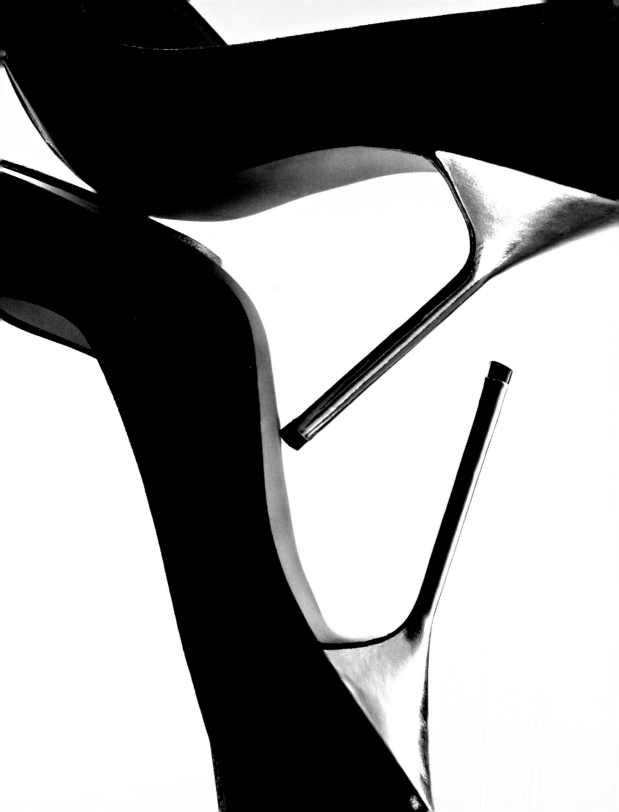

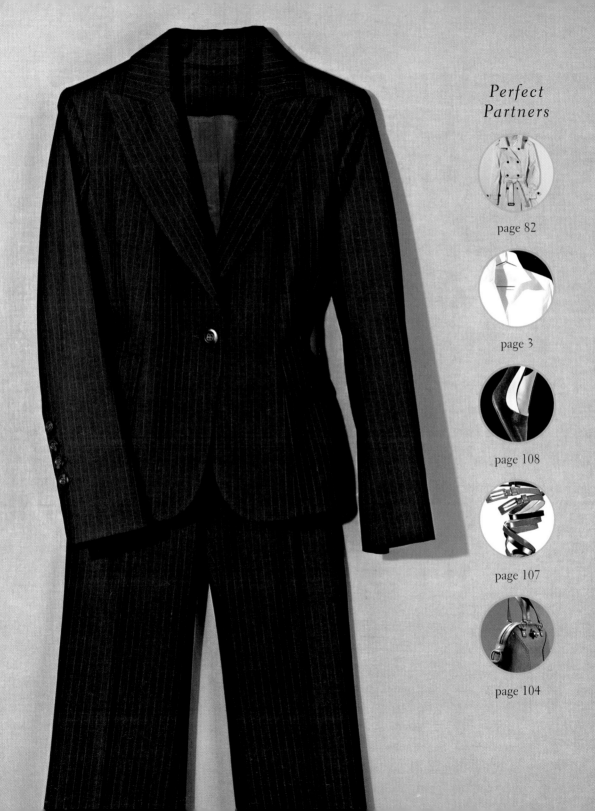

*Perfect
Partners*

page 82

page 3

page 108

page 107

page 104

Whether it brings to mind the stately look of *The Great Gatsby* or that of a gritty Hollywood gangster, the classic pin-striped suit will always stand alone as an instant indicator of eye-catching style. The striking visual pull of the long, graphic lines of the fabric's pattern works with the soft shape of a woman's figure. The bold lines unite shoulder with toe, creating an arresting fluidity of movement.

Don a pin-striped suit properly and onlookers won't be able to take their eyes off

THE PIN-STRIPED SUIT

you. Thus it's the perfect addition to a woman's business wardrobe.

Keep in mind that sharp suits such as this crave softer underpinnings to create a visual balance of his-meets-hers. And this yin-yang styling approach is easier than you might think. Here's this style expert's top ten list of unanticipated alternatives for any season.

FOR WEARING WITH	YOU MIGHT CHOOSE	TRY THIS INSTEAD
pin-striped jacket	crisp white shirt	satin blouse with ruffles
pin-striped skirt	sharp blazer	feminine sweater set
pin-striped pant	solid turtleneck	off-the-shoulder top
pin-striped jacket	tailored trouser	denim trouser
pin-striped skirt	blouse and sweater vest	T-shirt and leather jacket or T-shirt and men's suit vest
pin-striped jacket	straight skirt	fuller skirt and belt for jacket
pin-striped pant	V-neck sweater	tank and denim jacket
pin-striped jacket	summer pant	Bermuda shorts
pin-striped pant	sweater vest and blouse	men's suit vest and T-shirt
pin-striped skirt	shell and pumps	sleeveless turtleneck and boots

uess who's coming to dinner, breakfast, and everything in between? It *is* black, but it's not Sidney Poitier! Why, the black turtleneck, of course! Think of a black turtleneck as the Henry Clay of a fashionable wardrobe, the great compromiser, if you will. Here are twenty-five classic and foolproof outfit combinations including this most versatile item.

THE BLACK TURTLENECK

+ black trousers + black patent leather flats

+ white jeans + red kitten heels

+ gray wool skirt + black slingbacks + fishnets

+ jeans + red thin belt (atop turtleneck) + animal flats

+ chinos + black trench + white sneakers

+ black and white pin-striped trousers + nude pumps

+ camel wool shorts + black tights + knee boots

+ black satin ball gown skirt + metallic heels

+ pink twill pants + wide black patent belt and flats

+ cream cords + kelly green blazer + sandals

+ dark denim skirt + black patent riding boots

+ camel high-waist pants + wine pumps

+ jeans + camel blazer + bright rubber wellies

+ white cotton pants + silver cuff + nude flats

+ taxi yellow cords + black velvet "jean" jacket

+ black satin pants + gold metallic heels

+ black and white floral skirt + yam kitten heels

+ black and white polka-dot capris + grass green flats

+ crisp white shirt (open) + jeans + sandals

+ camel leather pants + gold cuff and hoops

+ black leather pants + black ankle boots

+ tan cords + red wool blazer + patent loafers

+ black yoga pants + pink ballet flats

+ red capri pants + black and white checked flats

+ black leather skirt + black boots + fishnets

Perfect Partners

page 183   page 171   page 202   page 92   page 180

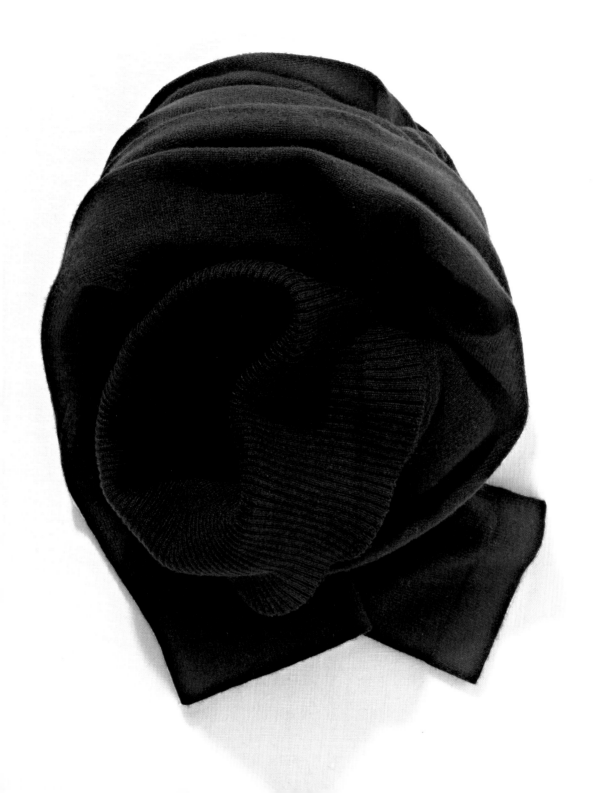

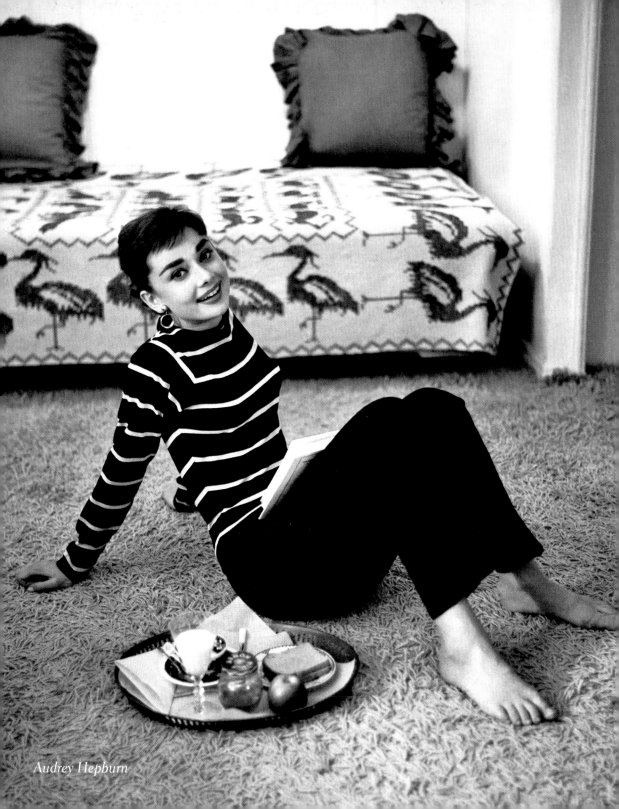
Audrey Hepburn

2 | WEEKEND

A roomy, go-to jean that welcomes you in, leg by leg, with no resistance, no judgment on what size you currently are, and no anxiety when it comes time to fasten that oft scary top rivet. Whew! It clasps with no strain—and actually offers the feeling that dessert is a real option today. This is a true easy jean. It is your best friend on days off, when worn with your best loose sweatshirt and jeweled flip-flops, or for days "on," combined with a smartly fitted blazer, sexy heels, and a satin camisole.

THE EASY JEAN

Now, with that said, a few things that easy jeans are *not*. They are not what some call "mom jeans." This denim pant can easily pass for an acid-wash eighties music video costume, boasting a waistband that can fall closer to your bust than your waistline. The mom jean makes your butt look longer and flatter than it actually is because of its tall pockets and super-high-rise waistband.

Here are three simple ways to narrow down the many options, especially when searching for an easy jean to add to your repertoire of weekend bottoms.

SEARCH OUT DENIM *TROUSERS* (NOT THE AVERAGE JEAN) Most labels offer jeans, the traditional four-to-five-pocket fitted pant style that we all know and love. Many of your favorite labels offer what are called denim trousers: pants constructed of denim but tailored in a dress-pant silhouette.

CROSS INTO *HIS* TERRITORY Easy jeans aren't called "boyfriend jeans" for naught! There was a time when girls couldn't find loose, easy bottoms—especially in denim. So they borrowed them from the closet of any male that they could because jeans cut for guys are usually fuller through the leg and thigh and looser at the highest point of the waist, and were traditionally more "broken in."

If the denim you're trying on makes you feel squeezed in, there is nothing wrong with shopping the men's section of your favorite store. You don't have to sentence yourself to the skintight low-riding hip-hugger britches of the 1970s that, as the Ohio Players sang, ran "folks into ditches."

SIZE UP AND STRETCH Keep in mind that denim even *without* a touch of stretch or Lycra in the fabric will loosen up and stretch out over time. If you really want total ease, buy them in your true size—or a size larger even. Just be sure that they fit and flatter around your hips and backside. A good tailor can work wonders on jeans too, if, in fact, your sized-up jeans need a little help in certain areas—such as the waistline—*before* you begin to wash and wear.

Perfect
Partners

page 78

page 37

page 33

page 202

page 205

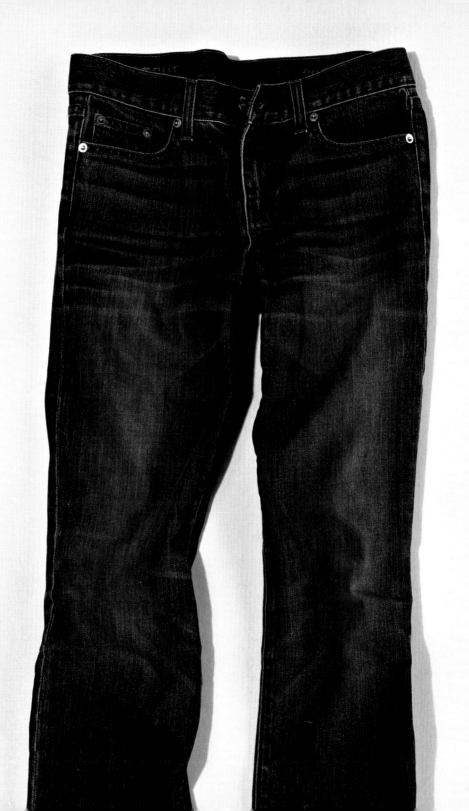

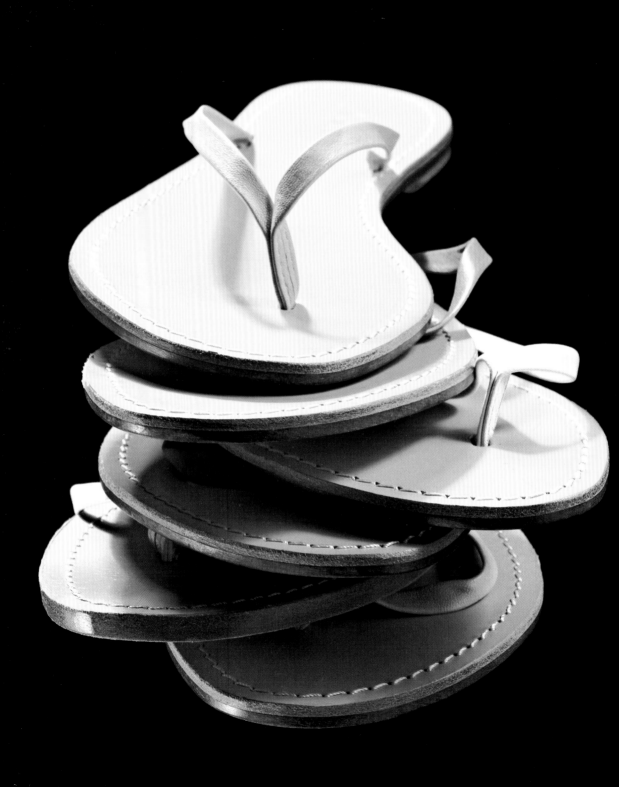

The thong sandal has become the poster child for the carefree look. And the rubber flip-flop, its cheaper little sister, is a benchmark of the same carefree look—turned care*less*.

Warmer months and generally warmer climates allow women to expose their tootsies with (sometimes reckless) abandon. And that's as it should be, for there may not be a better feel-

THE THONG SANDAL

ing than a breeze over and between the toes as you enjoy a beautiful day outdoors. But are your feet and sandals ready for their close-up?

The right thong sandal should be magical! It should offer you the comfort you crave, style you would envy on the foot of another well-dressed woman, and that perfect finishing touch to a casual outfit. A flesh-toned rendition is usually the best first investment.

This magic happens on versions that boast leather soles, perfectly finished stitching details on the thong and sole, and a design that speaks of something special (metallic-finish leather; faux-jewel-encrusted details; an intense color, print, or pattern). All of a sudden, your easy, kick-around shoes become kicky and unique—and able to stand alone, complementing just about anything, like a good animal-print accessory.

Most stylists would agree that they would rather women owned two or three amazingly chic, well-crafted thong sandals than dozens of inexpensive rubber flip-flops that look as if you just left the spa with a pedicure. Taking the time to find these ideal additions is a journey that should be fun, not frustrating. If you find them too quickly, or for a steal, they *may* not be the best for your footwear collection.

Sometimes you get lucky, but if the pair you consider is hanging fastened together on a plastic hook and being sold in a rainbow of colors right in between the sunscreen and the Styrofoam coolers, buyer beware!

Perfect Partners

page 34   page 30   page 122   page 74   page 217

Whether you have a man in your life or not, a menswear shirt is something you can always have and hold. What makes it so sexy is the fact that it is not traditionally meant for a feminine frame. The contrast is what creates the real sexiness. Take a look at eight tried-and-true ways to feature a menswear shirt for any occasion.

THE MENSWEAR SHIRT

FOR THE OFFICE Of course you could wear it beneath a pantsuit. But wear it untucked with your sexiest pencil skirt, vixen heels, and a wide or slim belt on top and go from boring to banging. Cuff the sleeves once—and finish off the look with back-seam stockings or nude fishnets.

FOR THE WEEKEND Buy it loose, easy, roomy, and even a size or two larger—this transforms *his* shirt into *her* best friend. Layer it on top of a fitted camisole in the same color. Combine it with cropped, flat-front khakis and your coolest flats in a jewel tone. Pass the Sunday paper, please!

FOR GIRLS' NIGHT OUT When all your girlfriends are skipping dessert in their fitted tops and slinky dresses, guess who's having (and enjoying) the crème brûlée? Select a solid black shirt usually meant for him, and style it for *her* by tucking it into your chicest dark jeans—but only buttoning the bottom button to start the evening. Pop the collar way up, and grab a shimmery evening clutch and strappy high heel for accents. A black lace camisole is the foundation. As the food and drinks add up, you simply button up!

FOR TRAVEL Grab his shirt in white. Grab your jeans or cords in white. And now grab your comfiest flats in red or orange! With the help of a gauzy linen scarf in white, you are done! Excuse me, miss, shouldn't you be in first class?

Perfect Partners

page 77   page 41   page 205   page 78   page 202

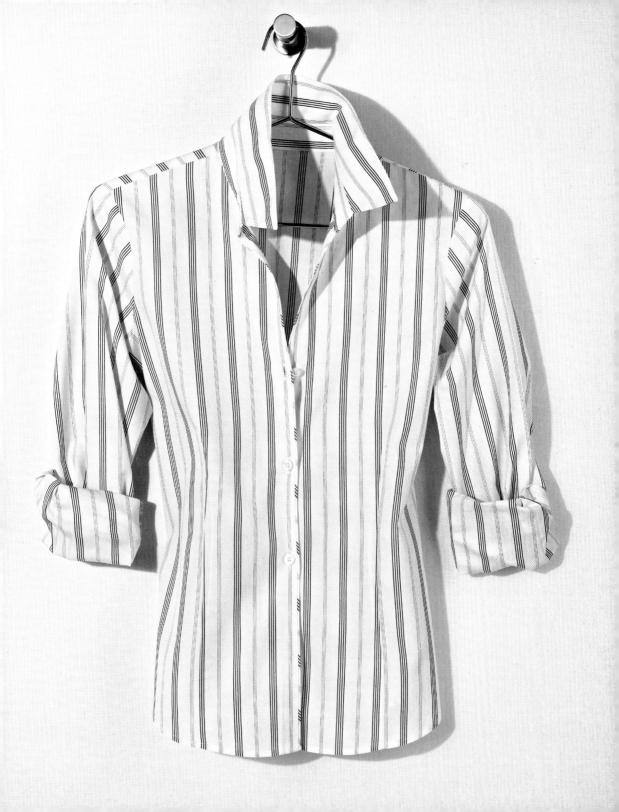

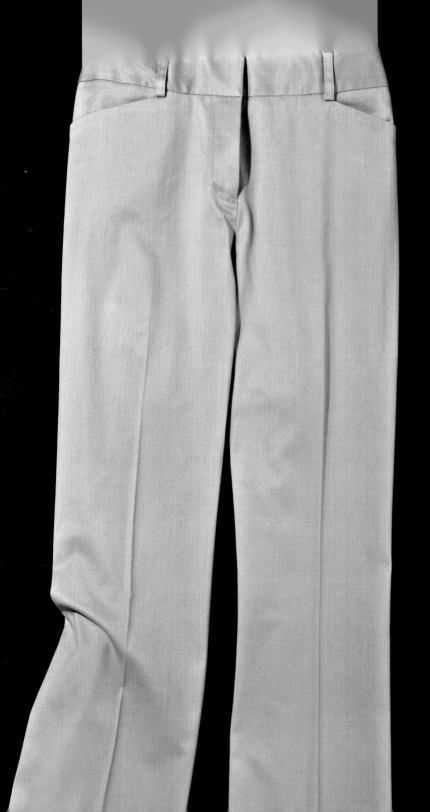

Perfect Partners

page 117

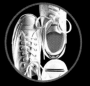

page 121

page 113

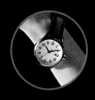

page 96

page 205

Some call them chinos, some call them a near year-round jean replacement—especially when a comfortable outfit needs a softer visual touch than the deep blue denim can provide.

Khakis originated in India in 1845 as British military men drenched their traditional white uniforms in coffee, curry powder, and mud in an effort to blend into the natural landscape. Fast-forward to 1912, when they made their United States debut on the bottoms of naval aviators. By the early 1930s, they could be found on the personnel manning sub-

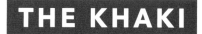

THE KHAKI

marines, and a decade later the navy approved khakis for on-station wear, but only by senior officers. It is said that Pearl Harbor chiefs and officers were the first to be authorized to wear khakis ashore on leave.

They are the coolant to almost any strong style essential you pair them with. Think of it as a nice big ice cube resting in a single-malt scotch, easing its strength, adding layers, notes, and texture with each sip. So many outfits rely on khakis to "chase" a stringent top or jacket.

Your khakis will do the same when you wear them with anything from the casual lace tank and denim jacket to a sharp black leather racing jacket and matching black sleeveless turtleneck.

The fit is critical, so be sure to locate the most modern versions that offer a smidge of stretch or Lycra (to help prevent wrinkles), pockets that lie flat to the body (to prevent bulging and lumps through the lightweight fabric), and tab-front closures without pleats (lending themselves to a more modern look, done dressy or casual). Let the hem skim the floor to be worn with your sexiest heels, and consider investing in a duplicate pair that you can hem just for flat shoes or sandals.

W eekend getaways are the stuff of legend. For decades, we have seen dreamy television commercials and glossy print ads that feature that "perfect" gorgeous couple throwing caution to the wind, gassing up the convertible, and tossing a great bag in the backseat before they ride off into the sunset.

THE WEEKEND BAG

A chic weekend bag is just as much a part of the getaway experience as your flirty dress for cocktails later that night. So make it special. All you need is one. You will feel so much better toting your belongings in that old gym duffel bag, canvas tote, or heavy rolling suitcase.

STYLE HAS ITS BENEFITS If you happen to be staying at a hotel, from the first bellman and concierge to the check-in representative and beyond, your style and the bag you carry will dictate the type of welcome you receive, almost as much as the price of your room.

So walking into a chic hotel for a weekend getaway dragging tattered, outdated luggage really says, "Please check me in as quickly as possible and get me out of this lobby to my standard room." Whereas on the other hand, the well-dressed woman who enters with just one impossibly fabulous weekender in her hand visually says, "Upgrade me to a suite, and give me a free cocktail while I linger in this stately lobby." I think she's starting a seriously memorable weekend—all with the help of a killer bag! Trust me.

FREQUENT USE IS A GOOD THING Just like a passport that has clearly seen many a global port judging by the pastiche of multicolored stamps on its pages, your investment-quality weekend bag will gain its own patina as you use it. If you choose leather it will bruise a bit here and there and boast a new texture over time—kind of like little travel badges of honor. Or your suede bag might take on swipes of your own body oil that give it a suntanned look of its own, speaking of jaunts to Aspen or the Alps. Either way your investment bag will get better with age.

Perfect Partners

page 51

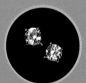

page 56

page 85

page 59

page 214

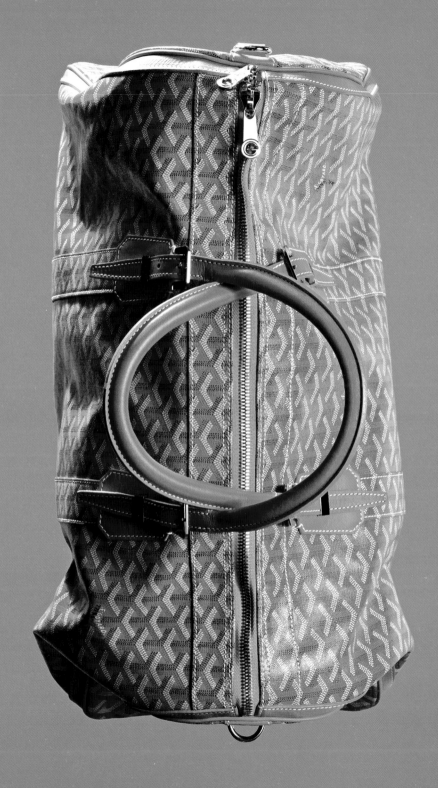

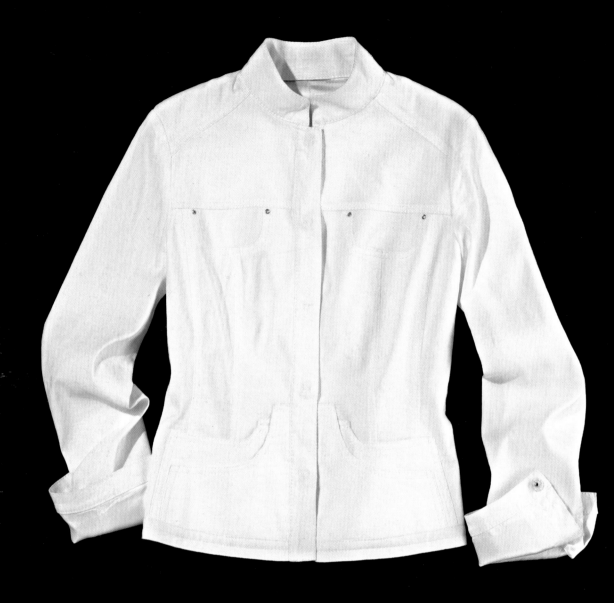

Perfect Partners

page 147   page 140   page 3   page 74   page 217

Although denim jackets have been around for well over one hundred years, they remain a huge part of "new" clothing collections each and every season. Some luxury designers offer a dressy version, keeping the more western-styled "jean jacket" shape and details but leaving the denim part behind—creating

THE WHITE DENIM JACKET

them out of black satin, for example. Other mass brands will add a faux-fur collar, which Old Navy made famously affordable, offering women a safe touch of chic to its legendary comfort.

Today, the *white* denim jacket is for all seasons. Check this off your style list and watch your chicness multiply.

WINTER White in winter? Absolutely! If the fabric stands up to colder weather, what should the color matter? Women who choose white clothes against the gray backdrop of winter always stand out in a fashionable way. Your white denim jacket makes your navy blue pin-striped suit pants look fresh and hip again. Layer in a solid navy blue turtleneck, silver accessories, and black suede shoes and satchel.

SPRING The jacket is great with grass green, like good fries scream for ketchup! Envision your jacket with a grassy green skirt, heather gray T-shirt, nude heels, and straw clutch. The look is fresh, flirty, and youthful.

SUMMER As it heats up outside, the world inside usually gets cooler thanks to the omnipresence of air-conditioning. That summer work dress in any color you choose now has a hipper shoulder-warmer.

FALL Of course you could purchase an indigo denim jacket, but why line up with the legions of other women who will do the same? Choosing a bleach-white version (in a style that is slightly less rebellious than the classic four-pocket western style) will assist you in creating outfits that speak to a more modern take on sporty autumn style. Denim fabrics can be applied to safari jackets and blazer hybrids, or even styled to look like zip-front racing jackets. Take the time to find the silhouette that works for *your* body. You will know it instantly when you try it on. When you do, make the fall your time to work it for all that it is worth, for the crisp air is a perfect match to a lightweight denim jacket—with anything *but* denim on the bottom. Combine it with corduroys in earth tones, add a knit top in a bright color, and finish the look with a long gauzy scarf and clutch bag. Good-bye pumpkin picking, hello art gallery opening!

*W*hat would summer be without the classic short-sleeve polo shirt? The answer is beyond simple. A boiling mess!

Today, you could walk into your favorite family discount store at the top of the summer not only to stock up on your outdoor entertaining essentials and sunscreen, but also

THE SHORT-SLEEVE POLO

to find a rainbow of stylishly fitted, soft-to-the-touch,

classically designed polo shirts. And not the frumpy, boxy versions of old inspired by their original model—those worn by professional male polo players.

Embrace the perfect short-sleeve polo like it is your warm-weather uniform. I suggest this top ten list for purchase in order of importance:

COLOR	TO WEAR WITH	INSIDER TIP
white	anything, all summer long	Nab two: one dressy, one casual.
black	black capris or shorts at night	Wash in cold water to keep noir.
navy blue	seersucker shorts or white pants	Amazing under a white blazer.
grass green	navy or white shorts and yellow flats	Just screams summer and youth.
orange	pink shorts or pants à la the sixties	Orange adds a sun-kissed glow.
hot pink	madras plaid shorts	Layer on a jean jacket to cool down.
yellow	pale gray bottoms of any kind	Summer is suddenly sophisticated.
turquoise	lightweight jeans or denim shorts	Bright ribbon belts will add punch.
a shocker	anything neutral on the bottom	An unexpected hue = visual heat!

Perfect Partners

page 26   page 147   page 205   page 202   page 206

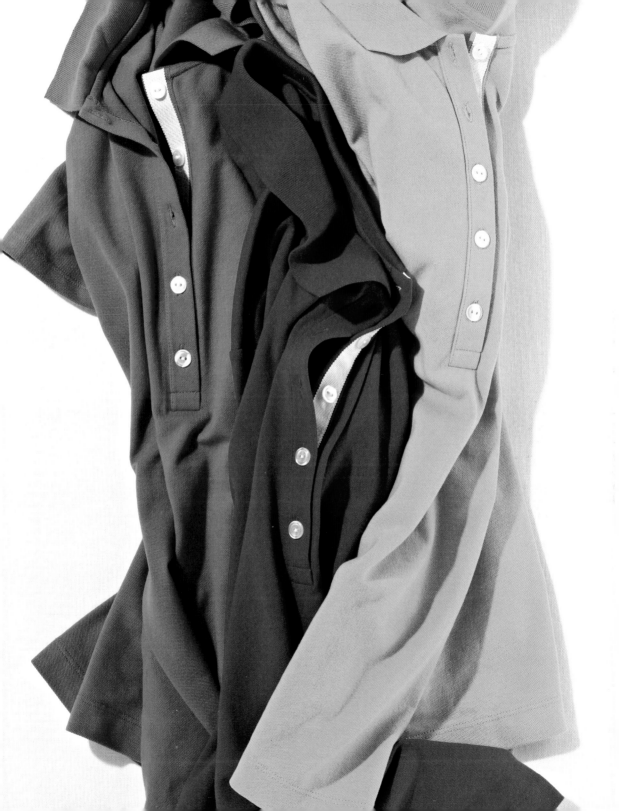

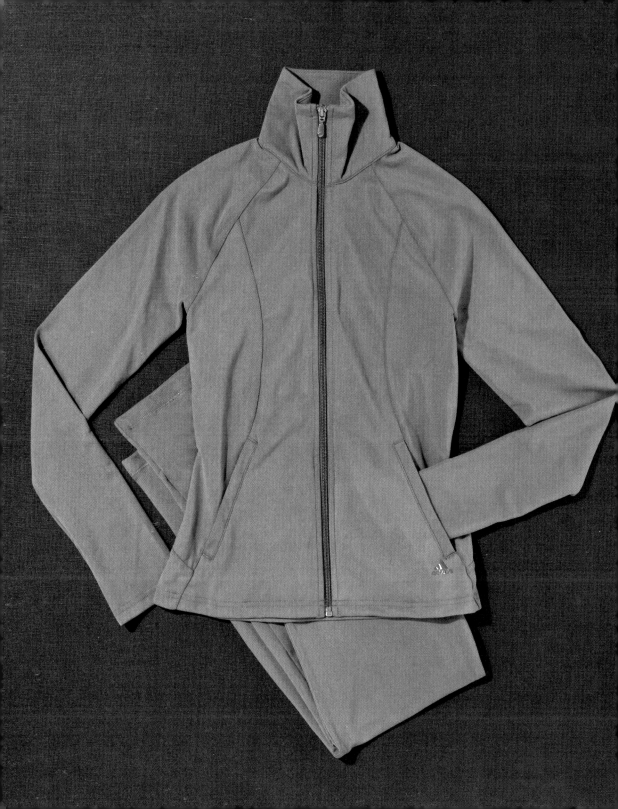

s it stylish? Not so much. Is it comfortable? Oh, yes! Does it have a place in the closet of a modern, stylish woman? This is for you to decide, after you read this.

WHAT WORKS Sometimes being chic isn't about what you wear but more about what you *avoid*.

WHEN TO MOVE ON Trends have a shelf

THE TRACKSUIT

life. An athletic classic for warming up/working out, the trend of the comfy, cozy tracksuit made an appearance among everyday clothes in the late 1970s (remember terry cloth?), early 1980s (remember velour?), and the late 1990s (remember the "Juicy" butt logo?), and held its ground well into the new millennium. And although Juicy Couture's signature tracksuit is still a part of their core brand, the company now offers everything from chic dresses and fragrance to menswear, kids' fashion, home goods, bags, and shoes. They have moved on from the tracksuit as king. "Butt" have you?

THE KEY Own a tracksuit; don't let it own *you*. Many women are afraid to break up their cozy companions. Oprah herself asked me in front of her millions of viewers if it was ever okay to wear them. The higher the quality, the better your chances of passing off the pants as a separate, making the perfect partner for a casual blazer, tank, and fun flat shoe. Or take the track jacket and layer it beneath a slim, quilted vest, add a sporty camisole, a denim miniskirt with tights, and wellie boots for a chic take on a chilly outdoor day look.

A STYLE BREATHER The tracksuit is best when you need a day *off* from style. Any woman who thinks she has to be well put together and chic each and every day of the calendar year is probably more stressed than the average gal. You need days off so your days *on* can feel special again. Don't make wearing the garment a way of life.

Perfect Partners

page 125   page 122   page 74   page 214   page 202

The white jean is a new classic of modern, casual dressing. Pure, fresh, simple, this closet classic can be the primer for just about any look that requires an infusion of crispness and light. And unlike the blue jeans that most women never think twice about incorporating into an outfit, the white jean is more feminine and not as limited as, let's say, indigo denim. While the blue

THE WHITE JEAN

washes of denim usually disappear in the eyes of others, white jeans vanish even faster and can work in limitless ways—and all year long. Don't be afraid to size them up and/or reserve them for outfits that have hip-grazing tops. Take a look at these four styling examples that work for every size and every season.

WINTER DISAPPEARING ACT Yes, white for winter! White denim, that is. Denim works all year long. The white jean is brilliant with a black velvet blazer, crisp white button-down shirt, and black boot! A touch of modern equestrian, and a whole lot of chic!

SPRING INTO MODERN NAUTICAL Your navy blue business suit jacket or a classic navy blue blazer with your bleach white jean will give you a hint of maritime mystique. This classic seaworthy combo yearns for shoes and tops in classic red, rain-slicker yellow, grass green, or gray heather. You can even mix two of the aforementioned colors to pop your navy and white nautical duo.

SUMMER NIGHTS DONE RIGHT Think Los Angeles. Think Milan. Think Paris! Wherever you draw your style inspiration from, the white jean can be a nighttime staple in these stylish cities. The trick is to never clutter the jean with overly wrought-out tops and shoes. They're best with shoulder-baring slip tops in juicy colors, and the sexiest of high heels or sparkly flats. Put your lip gloss and a fresh, summery scent on and you're out the door. Done!

LEGENDS OF THE FALL When most women run to their dark jeans, toasty-toned cords, and chino bottoms, the woman who gets *good* stares rocks a beautifully fitted pair of white jeans. This style expert loves them with almost any fall topper, from a nubby hand-knit poncho to a military-inspired peacoat in just about any dark or jewel tone, even. The jean softens while *stabilizing* your outerwear so you don't look like you have on head-to-toe cold-weather gear—at least not just yet. There's plenty of time to fight the bulky "Michelin woman" look looming in months ahead. Use the fall season to balance the look of your bulkiest tops and coast with the foundation of a lean, crisp white jean.

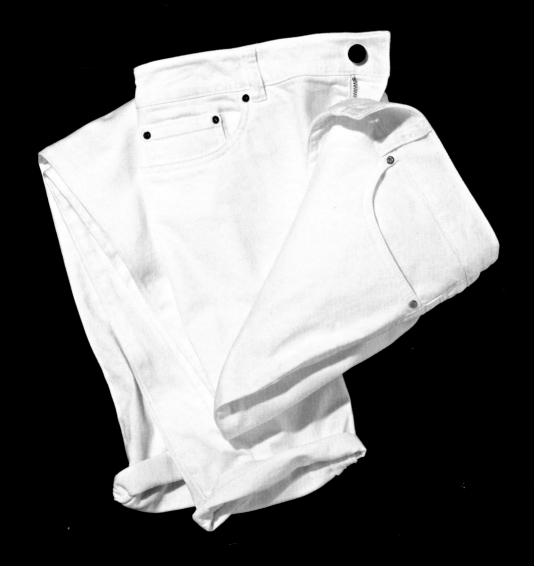

Perfect Partners

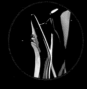

page 55   page 48   page 166   page 201   page 206

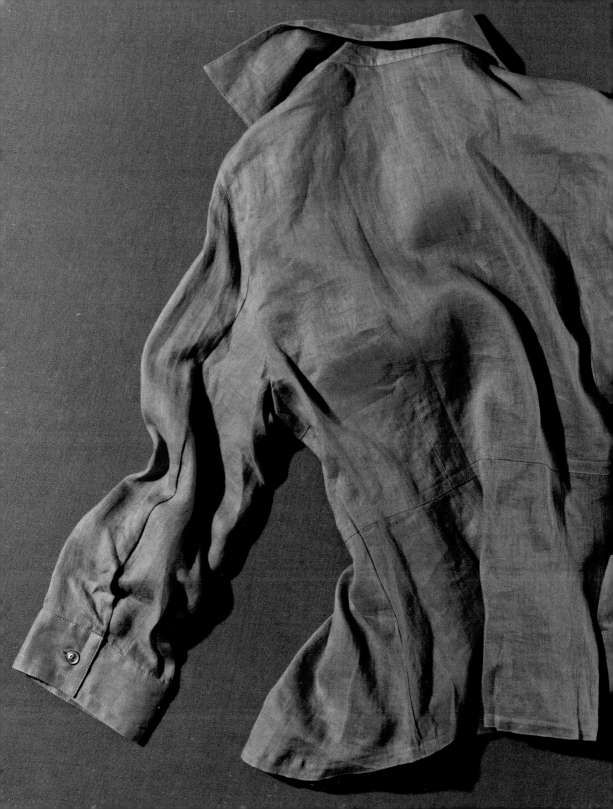

When most women are trying to avoid wrinkles at any cost, well-dressed women willingly embrace them, at least in one area of their lives—owning a fetchingly rumpled linen shirt!

A cornerstone of summer style, the linen shirt is still on the receiving end of style discrimination. I can't count the num-

THE LINEN SHIRT

ber of times that I have recommended a beautiful linen garment to a woman I am shopping with, only to have her instantly and emphatically say, "Oh, no! That's lovely, but it's *linen*. It will wrinkle." As if that's the only fabric that wrinkles.

The linen shirt is to the starched, pressed cotton shirt what a handwritten letter on beautiful parchment paper is to an email that takes seconds to send. It remains a nostalgic, romantic take on the easiest way to start a stylish summer ensemble that looks like you weren't trying at all.

A white, 100 percent Irish linen shirt is the first step; then add other colors and prints. Keep four important things in mind about this fabric's unique texture.

IT IS WHAT IT IS—BEAUTIFUL Linen's natural tendency to wrinkle only *adds* to its charm. Each time you wear it, you will discover a different flow of the lines and furrows. Try seeing it from a fresh point of view so you can really own it and work it!

IT LOVES A SMOOTH PARTNER Ultra-wrinkled items, including the linen shirt, look amazing when worn with bottoms that have a clean, smooth finish—such as a sharp skirt that hugs your curves (in a stretch-infused fabric that *resists* wrinkles). This pairing will highlight the beauty of the shirt, giving it a strong stage to show its movement and textural qualities and deflect the spotlight onto the smoother bottom.

Perfect Partners

page 30

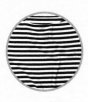
page 113

page 26

page 33

page 96

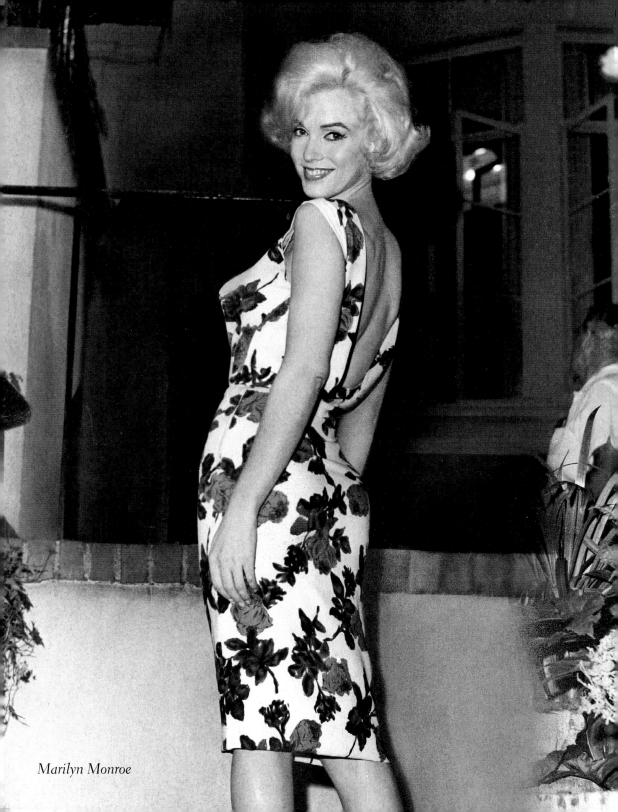

Marilyn Monroe

3 | SATURDAY NIGHT

What exactly is a party dress? Is it a frock that comes complete with the hope of a fun get-together attached? Is it a gown replete with all the makings of a sparkly night already built in? The answers should be yes!

In the 1950s, the party dress was a special-occasion dress that was created of fancier fabrics like satin or silk—versus your everyday dresses of wool or cotton. Today's party dress is very differ-

THE PARTY DRESS

ent. Today's hippest designers are creating it in washed embroidered silk, which gives an easy, youthful look to a once precious fabric. Animal-printed jersey is another favorite that won't cling as you dance, flirt, or discreetly prowl. And even poly/rayon/spandex blends can now look elegant—if you choose the right label (hint: Tracy Reese). If the party is more conservative or businesslike, the appropriate dress may cover the knee and have a higher neckline, offering even less cleavage and décolletage. When the occasion is not about business and, let's say, means dancing, the dress becomes eye candy.

Fitting in is fine, but standing out is what gave many of the world's real "party girls" their moniker. Flipping the script makes the party secondary to you; the best-dressed guest inspires others to have even more fun. The most important points when selecting the standout dress are the perfect fit, a fabric or pattern that looks like you want to touch it from across the room, a color that stands alone amid a sea of expected little black dresses, and a design that puts your *best* assets on a silver platter (without looking like you are trying!).

The trick is to nearly reverse the theme of the night wherever you decide to party! Go against the expected grain and distinguish yourself as a woman of style. When shopping for your party look, scan the racks, boutiques, or stores that you'd otherwise pass. And just like films in the 1930s, your wardrobe will all of a sudden go from black and white to Technicolor. This is when the real party begins! And it all starts with one unpredictably unique dress.

The one major thing *not* to do when selecting a party dress? Never put fashion before fit. Allow yourself the courtesy of choosing the size that fits (not the size you hope to be), and complete the investment with the help of a professional tailor for a truly polished finish.

Perfect
Partners

page 73

page 217

page 161

page 188

page 214

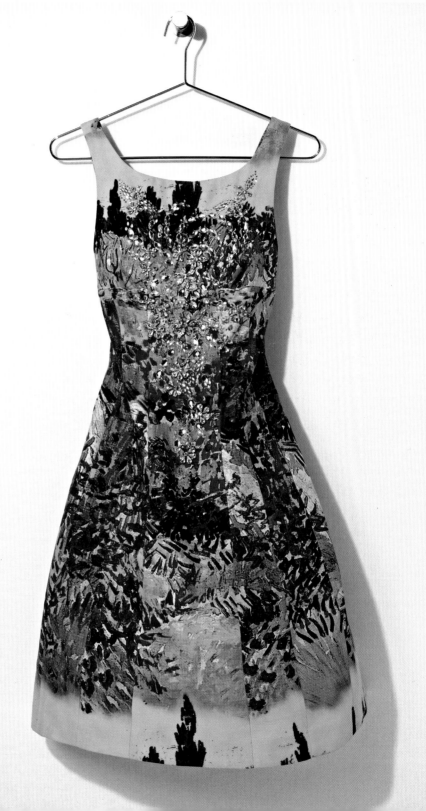

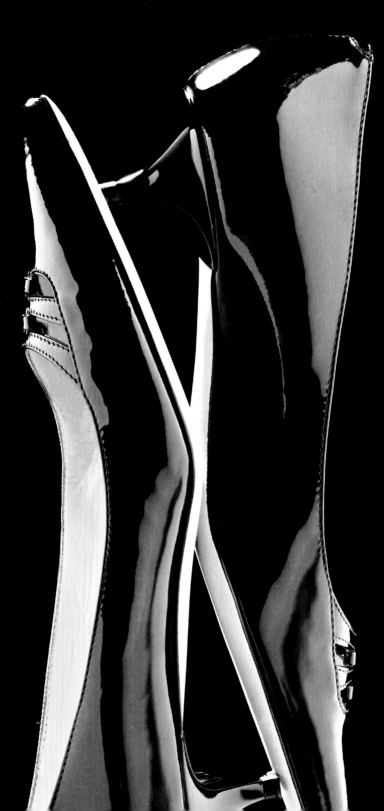

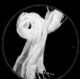
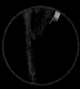

s there such a thing as sensibly chic heels? For many women this is not an oxymoron and the answer is a resounding yes!

The best stylists know that the key to a fantastic look is balance. For instance, if your top is shoulder-baring and designed for the truly body confident, your bottom of choice ought to be anything besides a skintight legging or short skirt—if you

THE SENSIBLY CHIC HEELS

aim to get *good* stares. The low heel is the perfect mix of both the top and bottom for spot-on visual balance.

If your cocktail dress is something safely sleeved, it could also be the appropriate chemise for the good girl in you to wear to church. But if you're doing the bad girl thing, rev up the heat for the night out by adding sultry slingbacks and a bold cherry lip. On the day after you can pair it with dark opaque tights and keep your lip color nude. The sensibly chic heel is something the good or bad girl can rock.

Look at the heels of shoes *first* when you shop, to identify the most artfully crafted sensible heels for your collection. A very slight curve always wins over the thick heel with little contour. The most petite and delicate top piece (the little stopper at the bottom of the heel that supports all your weight) looks best when it is smoothly flush and sculpted without interruption from the seat (or top) of the heel down. And last, the heel breast (the somewhat hidden *inside* of the heel that faces forward with you) must look as finished as the sides of the heels that face the world. You'd be surprised at how and where cheap manufacturers decide to cut corners, only to give away your spending secrets when you cross your legs—and you never quite know why the other women in the room are a little amused.

Today, more than ever, comfortable can also mean chic and affordable. Brands and designers alike are boasting affordable luxury to women everywhere—you just have to look and know when to balance your bargains with bits of pure decadence. The perfect low heel will do both and allow you to be the last woman standing, and dancing even.

F aye Dunaway famously posed for *Vogue* magazine's Jerry Schatzberg in 1968 in a cropped, button-front leather jacket and signature beret, channeling her film role as the infamous 1930s gangster Bonnie Parker, Clyde Barrow's other half. The leather jacket craze continued into the 1970s as the garment was seen everywhere, including on the backs of Afro'd female Black Panthers, layered atop black miniskirts and knee boots. And how can we forget the 1980s,

THE LEATHER JACKET

when Cher got tough in her black leather motorcycle jacket for her "If I Could Turn Back Time" video. She paired it with nothing but a thong and an authentic white sailor's cap.

Leather jackets continue to rule. Consider what is most age appropriate in styling with leather, using inspiration from decades past for decades to come.

TWENTYSOMETHING Go for the leather trench in the most butter-soft leather you can find, in a color other than black. Think cognac, espresso, or mahogany. Toss it on with anything from your sexiest jeans to that delicate lace dress for a truly hip styling contrast.

THIRTYSOMETHING The blazer is best—in a black and at a paper-thin weight. You'll turn heads. Swap out your black suit's jacket, add a bold red lip, and pop your collar up to give the look an instant nighttime flair. Taxi!

FORTYSOMETHING Go full metal jacket on them! It could be cut in the manner of a racing jacket or mandarin style. Or even military. All of these silhouettes are timeless, as should be your style at this point. Choosing it in bronze, pewter, copper, or even gold will punctuate the fact that you really own your look and transcend trends that seduce your younger counterparts.

FIFTYSOMETHING AND BEYOND Make it short and sweet with a cropped leather jacket tapered at the waist that splits the hip, in a pale color. A zip-front version will taper your midsection when half-closed and make even your yoga pants ready for a ladies' lunch!

Perfect Partners

page 9   page 103   page 91   page 59   page 205

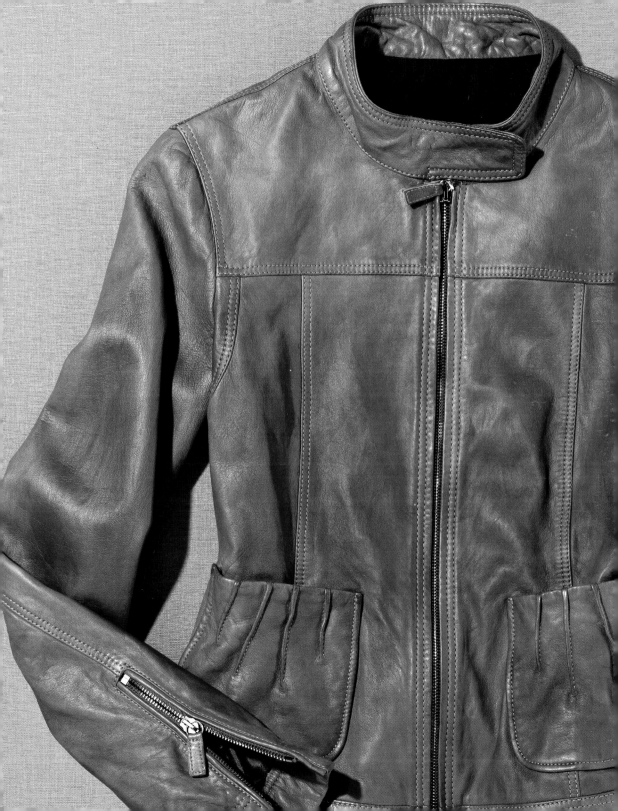

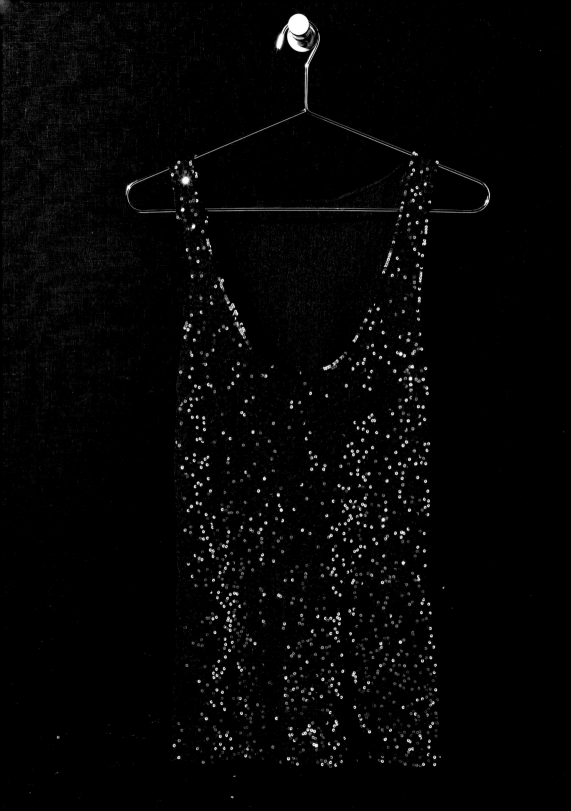

There are few clothing items that flatter almost *all* women of any shape, age, or size. Oddly enough, the sequined tank is one of them. Skinny girls can slink around in one, tossing it on with a pair of matchstick jeans done in satin or white denim. Curvy chicks might jump into one with a full, A-line skirt and a cropped jacket. And whether you are twentysomething or seventy-plus, the timeless elegance of sequined embellishment is something that keeps you looking youthful—without looking like you are trying to dress like the "youngins." It is a

THE SEQUINED TANK

"forever" garment that in proper measure says sizzle, dazzle, and sheen!

Layer it beneath anything from a denim jacket to a dark tailored man trouser. Let it give a glimmer of life from under a sleek, dark trench. Balance with a pencil skirt for creative business meetings or when going to "hot spot" dinners.

Choose sequins that look more matte and offer more luster and glow rather than brazen shine. Envision matte pewter, noir, copper, or bronze embellishments, artfully placed atop a matching tank in a feathery cashmere or silk. Or even high-gloss indigo sequins the size of nickels, whimsically placed upon a spaghetti-strap tank that *barely* hangs on your shoulders—this cheeky layering foundation is the start of a fun night, no matter where you are heading.

The sequined tank brings its own bling, serving as more of an *accessory* for the body than its plainer relations. As a consequence you don't have to add jewelry to the look. It brings attention to the most flattering focal point on a woman—her décolletage.

This garment adds a stately-meets-shimmery classic to your collection.

Perfect Partners

page 183   page 179   page 161   page 217   page 92

This blouse is a direct descendant of the signature chiffon handkerchief *dresses* made famous in the early 1900s by the famous French couturiere Madeleine Vionnet. She was a legend of innovative draping who inspired many contemporary designers such as Geoffrey Beene, Halston, and Issey Miyake. These and other top designers referenced the weightlessness of her bias-cut designs in dangerously sexy pieces that were calculatedly balanced with near impossible ease *and* taste.

THE SCARF BLOUSE

It's a top that parties with you when partnered with slimmer pants that allow its blouson-fit shape to shine, fluttering around your body as you dance, flit through a breezy room, or simply sit perched on a high stool for champagne. The design can also travel with you as the chicest, most unexpected swimsuit cover-up or top for shopping when slipped into a cool white pant or Bermuda short. And did I mention that it is beyond forgiving, especially when Mother Nature decides to drop off your monthly gift—if, that is, you are still on her list of rounds?

If there is ever a reason to take a hint from the past and bring it right into the present, it is when trends abound, threatening a clonelike copycat style pandemic. Now I have given you a secret weapon to combat the clones—and hopefully you have given yourself permission to wear it.

Perfect Partners

page 56

page 180

page 205

page 202

page 171

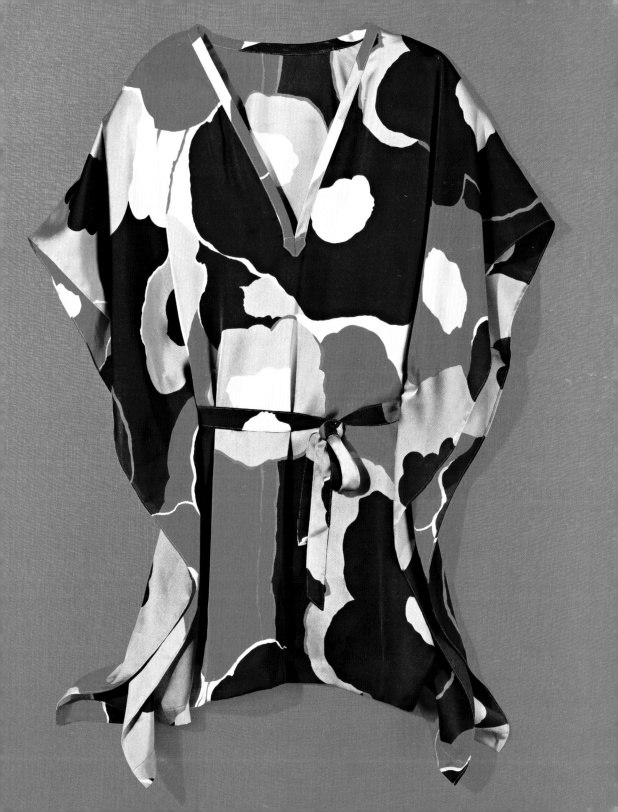

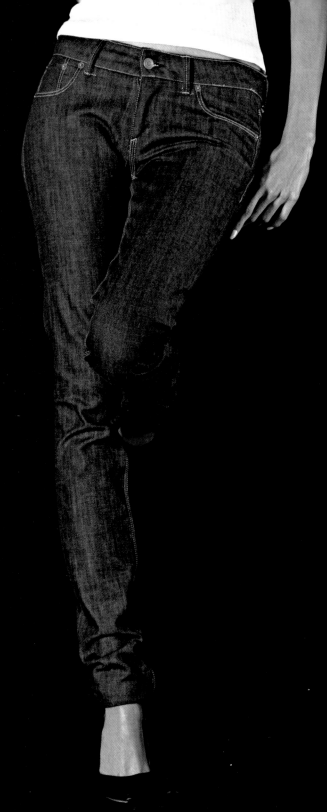

*Perfect
Partners*

page 162

page 59

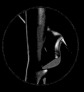

page 107

page 103

page 214

When you invest the time and money in discovering your perfect pair of traffic-stopping jeans, the style returns can be endless. And nowadays it usually requires more *time* than money, in that quality denim with a great fit and great details is available at so many price points. Long gone are the days when pricey "designer" denim options (that cost you more than a small car payment) were the only designs that actually fit and flattered.

THE TRAFFIC-STOPPING JEAN

If you take the time and enlist the help of a friend for a second opinion, one can find an amazing jean in your favorite mass retailer—or even online, if you don't mind the process of returning the pairs that don't fit. A small job in exchange for finding your true fit.

Here's how to wear your traffic-stopping jean at any juncture in your life.

TWENTYSOMETHING You are still the girl who has the legs that your older friends envy. Make sure the fit of your jeans drives this point home every time you jump into them. Pair them with super-slim heels and silky slip tops or basic men's tanks that look like you barely need a bra beneath them—while you can!

THIRTYSOMETHING The rinse should get slightly darker, and the fit should accommodate your now womanly lower half with a bit more room. Pair them with tops that hint at skin, but don't give it all away. There's nothing better than a hot dark jean tucked into a sexy leather knee boot and topped off with a fitted, sleeveless turtleneck (and a huge metal cuff on one arm). This is total runway chic. Add a fitted, cropped jacket to take the look right into casual evenings.

FORTYSOMETHING You have the super-sexy jeans and own enough sensible versions. Now it is time to embrace white jeans! Mix them with a fitted navy blue blazer and fun yellow patent leather flats for a feminine take on nautical—just add your favorite V-neck T-shirt. This decade allows you to light up the room without going the silly sexy route. You've earned it!

FIFTYSOMETHING AND BEYOND With a full collection of jeans that tell your life story in each style, where do you go now? I say luxury. A jean is merely a pant style that is most popular in a rugged cotton fabric most know as denim. But remember that you can treat yourself to jeans in midnight navy satin, plush tan moleskin, or even sandy linen for summer. I am sure your good old blues have served you well, and still will, but your new stretch black velvet version will make the holidays sparkle when paired with an untucked crisp white shirt, metallic kitten heels, and chunky necklace! Being called "grandma" just got a pushed a few years out.

A top-quality camisole is the perfect innerwear (and sometimes outerwear), a cousin to the bra. Most women know to own a few for longer coverage beneath tops, within dresses, or even under tailored jackets. Some spend a fortune on silky versions that require as much care as the dry-clean-only garments they undergird; others buy them for much less—and can wash them right along with their sporty T-shirts.

THE CAMISOLE

The choice is yours to make. The styling of the camisole is what's important, requiring us to think outside the tonal and predictable.

When investing in (or refreshing) your supply of camisoles, cover the bases by choosing a collection that goes from understated, to unexpected, to unforgettable!

CAMISOLE	UNDERSTATED BENEATH	UNEXPECTED BENEATH	UNFORGETTABLE BENEATH
Flesh-toned	matching top	low-cut white shirt	cream pantsuit
Black	black suit jacket	low-cut, bold-color caftan	leather jacket and sexy jeans
White or Ivory	floral dress	black blazer and walking short	white/ivory jeans and shrug
Lace	wrap top	menswear shirt	cropped jacket with shine
Matte-Metallic	navy blazer	black pant and black V-neck sweater	animal-print cardigan
Bold-Color	camel jacket and white shirt	low-cut black-and-white dress	dark denim jacket and pinstriped pants

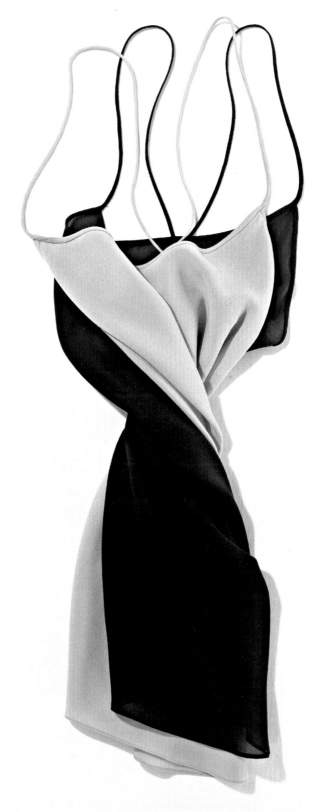

*Perfect
Partners*

page 81

page 41

page 17

page 64

page 217

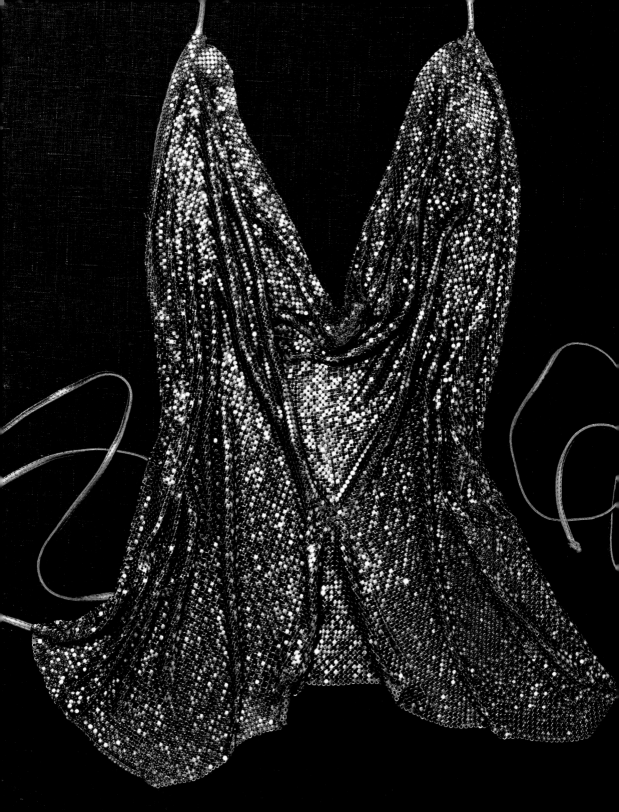

*S*elect a version that cradles your bustline tastefully, secures around the neck with total comfort, and floats away from your midsection with just enough room to forgive your dessert.

For you ladies who have fallen out of love with your arms, know that the halter top welcomes layering to conceal some parts of you and reveal others. For instance, a lightweight shrug that can shroud your arms allows for a hint of skin as it drapes open to slightly reveal the shoulder area. Or create a cheeky

THE HALTER TOP

take on an elegant evening look by adding an opera-length glove in a matching color that comes up to the elbow. Pop a cocktail ring atop your glove, and the look is an irreverent twist on the classics once reserved only for high-society evenings.

Another wonderful take on the halter top is a rendition that features built-in jewelry! Collars that have tiny rhinestones, tasteful monochromatic sequins all over, touches of ethnic beading, or simply a shimmery metallic fabric really do allow the wearer to leave all her jewelry in the box. They're not only a time-savers; these versions also speak to a modern woman who embraces the power of stylish restraint, leaving the overly baubled women in the dust. Again, less is modern.

Keep in mind that your arms will take center stage in a halter unless you choose to layer a wrap or covering over them. With this in mind, the tasteful equation begins with covering your lower stems a bit more. Try long skirts that flare around the lower leg and knee, a full A-line skirt, or pencil-straight cigarette pants that give the look of the 1960s (ladies with bold hips, beware). The best choice for curvy girls who love halter tops would be voluminous skirts à la the 1950s but updated a bit.

Any way you choose to don or alter your halter, know that you have two basic roads to take—uptown and sophisticated, or downtown and slightly edgy-sexy-chic! For isn't that the beauty of being a woman?

Perfect Partners

page 165   page 180   page 92   page 214   page 161

o you possess your own version of a dress that holds the power to unhinge an onlooker's jaw? If not, it's about time to use the power of a dress to feel strong, sexy, and unforgettable.

This style is meant to inspire you to not ever forget the power of the *sexiest* you. If you are ready to step on the gas and add this heat to your arsenal of style, here are the top three elements that deem a dress a jaw-dropping experience through and through.

THE JAW-DROPPING DRESS

FIT, FLATTERY, AND FORGIVENESS These are the good "F" words. You should know it right away. The dress fits your every curve with room to breathe. The color, pattern, or texture instantly flatters your skin, hair, and eyes. And the forgiveness happens without looking like you are trying to hide anything at all.

IT *FEELS* AS GOOD AS IT LOOKS Jaw dropping only ensues when your every step looks fluid, easy, and magical. Comfort is what makes this happen. That means first, being comfortable with your body; second, experiencing a fabric that caresses but won't cling (think silk, matte jersey, or stretch-infused fabrics); and last, having the comfort of knowing that no part of your dress will fall off.

IT IS SUPPORTED FROM THE INSIDE *OUT* Don't be afraid to add shaping undergarments, no matter your size. Even the slimmest woman can have a lump or two, which can ruin a sexy look. Ever heard of "skinny fat"? It's a real concern that justifies shapewear for women of all sizes.

Undergarment queen Rebecca Apsan, owner of La Petite Coquette, New York's premier destination for precise bra fittings and custom-fit lingerie, has a unique take on test-driving shapewear specifically, which most women overlook. "If it feels comfortable, the first thing you should check are the edges. Make sure your skin doesn't bulge where the *edges* of the fabric meet your body. You'll never get a smooth look under clothing if the garment simply *displaces* the problem bulges to other locations."

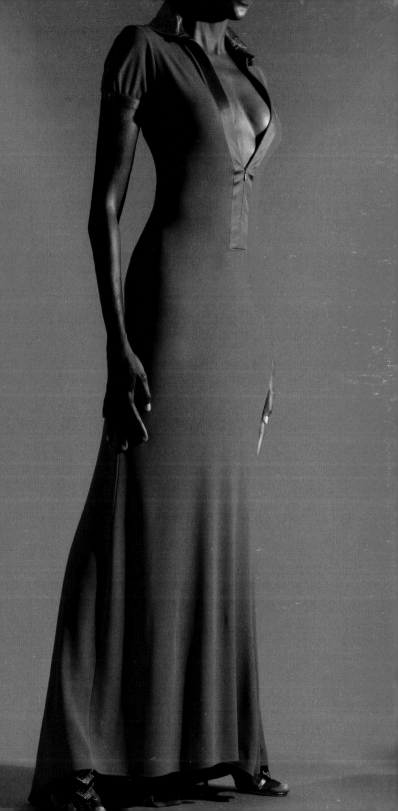

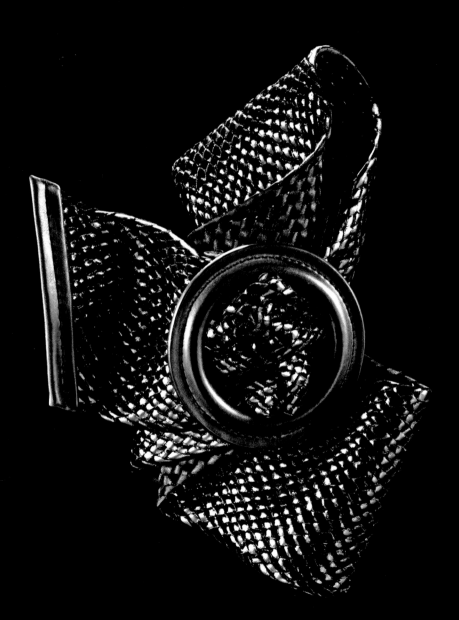

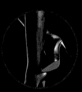

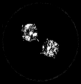

efore you start mentally shrilling about the waist you don't have or not knowing how to wear it, take a breather. You don't need as small of a waist as you might assume, and integrating it into your existing style skill set is simpler than you'd imagine, fun, and offers major style returns.

Peep these four unexpected ways you can make the wide belt work for *your* figure, style, and bank account all year round.

THE WIDE BELT

WINTER—FOR A QUICK WAY TO LOSE FIVE (VISUAL) POUNDS Got a black button-down shirt? How about a wide black belt in a stretchy material? If you have these two closet classics, all you need is a tailored pant or fitted skirt in any color known to man—and a great pair of heels. And whether you layer the belt atop the skirt, tucked, or use the belt to cinch the untucked shirt (using the shirttails to conceal the hips/backside), you will instantly have a leaner-*looking* upper half, especially amid that midwinter, post-holiday bloat.

SPRING—FOR A RETRO TAKE ON A NEW LOOK Spring's unpredictable weather shifts call for smart layering strategies. A three-part styling trick for making dresses look seventies cool all starts with your lightest-weight tank dress or shift, an even lighter crisp white blouse, and a wide belt. Layer the dress on top of the shirt, using it like a schoolgirl's jumper. Finish the look with a wide belt to secure the deal; this ensures that it looks mature, not middle school–ish.

SUMMER—GIVE YOUR HIPS SOME LOVE Summertime is meant for loose, gauzy, peasantlike tops that allow you to actually enjoy a backyard barbecue or poolside cocktail hour. You can do this without looking pregnant too! Add a wide belt in chain loops, woven macramé, or even a touch of hippie-inspired suede lanyards. Ignore your natural waist and let it rest atop one hip and sling low on the other.

FALL—FOR THE *NEW* BUSINESS CASUAL Take it from a fashion industry insider: You can belt almost any casual blazer or jacket and jolt it with a new energy. Imagine your favorite dark denim blazer paired with a tailored printed dress. The two might usually look at odds with each other. A stately wide belt in beautiful patent leather, a metallic faux animal skin (such as python or zebra), or just a simple fabric belt with a bold metal clasp will marry the two in perfect harmony. It will be the fashion translator of sorts.

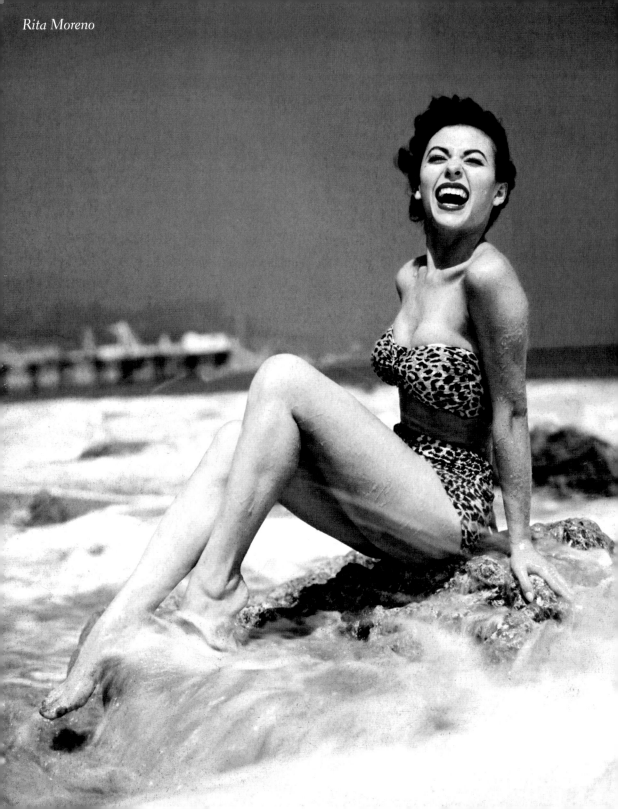

Rita Moreno

4 | TRAVEL

S tructure holds an important place in all well-curated closets. Strong lines; clean, sharp seams; and tailoring that offers linear impact to the eye add balance. Pieces that offer this rigidity are what allow your softer, flowing skirts, fuller pants, and frilly dresses to really shine as they were meant to.

THE SAFARI JACKET

One standout connector of the soft and structured sides of a well-dressed woman's closet is the safari jacket. Holding its post as a bona fide star on the list of wardrobe essentials, this tried-and-true design has been reinterpreted countless times since its midcentury women's fashion blessing by Dior. Heres how to wear it through *your* ages.

TWENTYSOMETHING Style it up with metallic aviator sunglasses, matchstick jeans (or *your* slimmest jeans) in a dark indigo rinse, and ankle boots. Cinch the self-belt if it still remains affixed, or add your own contrasting belt in patent leather or a fun faux snakeskin.

THIRTYSOMETHING Choose a version that can be a stand-in for the predictable suit jacket. A rendition in black or navy can make a matching work skirt feel more New York— regardless of where you work. Knee boots punctuate a skirt-and-safari-jacket duet.

FORTYSOMETHING A silk-and-linen-blend safari jacket is what your weekend cords, chinos, and casual business bottoms crave—but you might not know it. Layer just a simple tank or T-shirt in a bold color beneath it, and add kicky, colorful flats for easy-cum-chic weekends.

FIFTYSOMETHING AND BEYOND Traveling in high style will be simple when you begin with a black or crisp white safari jacket. Have fun with the material (leather, sateen, or even slick patent leather). If you select one in white, the fact that it is colorless means that it will marry well with anything you pack along with it.

Perfect Partners

page 183   page 59   page 33   page 48   page 202

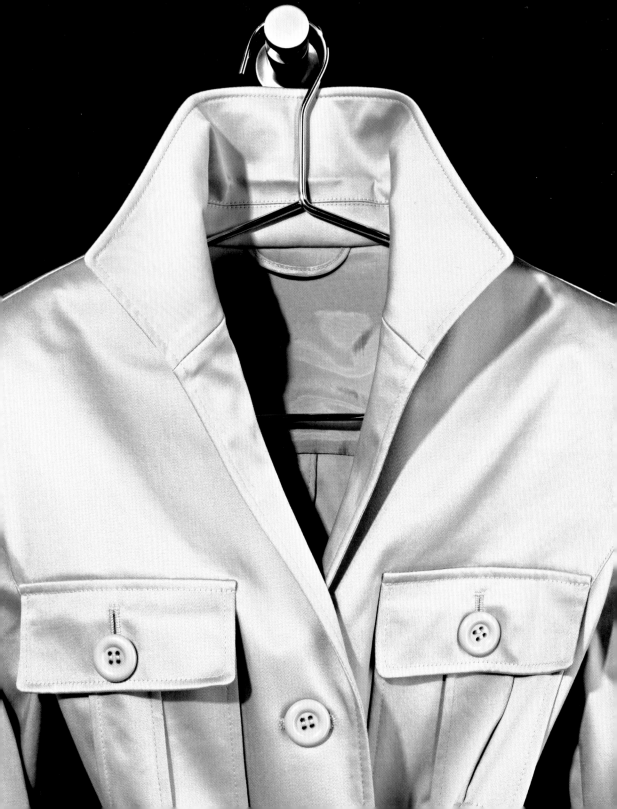

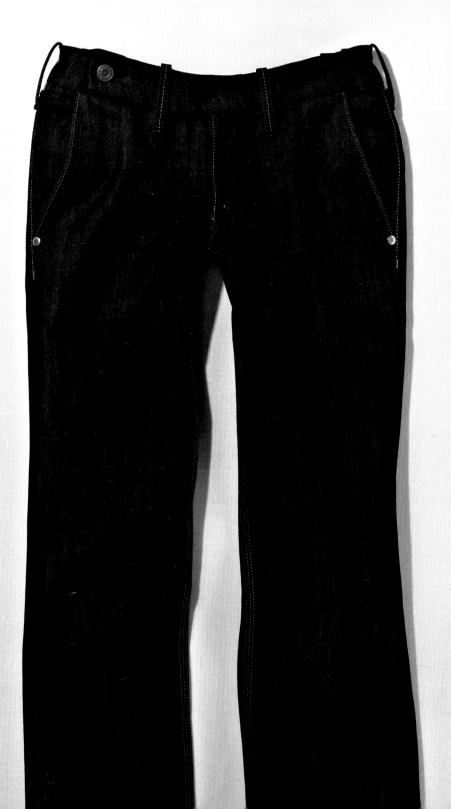

Perfect Partners

page 169

page 3

page 157

page 104

page 175

Although the riveted jeans we know today have been around since the mid-1800s, the trouser jean, which usually *doesn't* feature the more casual, westernwear-inspired riveting technique, became popular in the 1970s. This is the decade when working women began featuring the denim of the moment on everything from shoes and handbags to casual suits and even hats. Yikes!

The one category that we've seen pop in and out of fashion since

THE TROUSER JEAN

is the trouser jean, a trouser, in its design and tailoring, made of a stiffer dungaree fabric—usually fashioned best in a dark indigo rinse with no bleaching, fashion washing, or distressing. The reason is that it combines the comfortable, casual feeling that jeans bring to the body with the appropriateness of a pant that is more common in the casual workplace, a pretty genius pairing. And traveling is a cinch, especially when your trouser jean assists you like a power executive assistant thinking ahead of you. It works with suit blazers when it's time to cool them down after meetings, or with your strappy metallic heels when it's time to hit the jazz clubs.

It's power doesn't stop there either. The trouser jean converts from the office to any outing without hesitation—unlike your more fitted, relaxed, or sexy jeans. If chosen properly, they should slightly float around the leg, fit a little closer around the hip and upper thigh, and have just enough space for a finger around the waist (allowing for tops to be easily tucked in or smoothly rest atop the waist). A subtly flared leg gives the pant its slack-like finish and can flatter a multitude of figures, from petites (who should get them as long as possible) to curvy gals (who should select pairs with wider waistbands to visually taper thicker waists).

The trouser jean is the ultimate entertaining or party pant! Why? Because it moves with you on the dance floor, punctuating your every dip, even if the dance floor turns out to be your living room rug. It leaves a little something to the imagination when you couple it with a sexier, fitted top. And most important, the trouser jean can smarten up an entire outfit for women of a certain age who are trying to avoid the look of their sixteen-year-old relatives in the latest "it" jeans.

Not only is this bottom a wise investment, boasting more style ROI than most other casual cotton bottoms, but based on what style editors have seen on the runways since the 1970s, it's not going anywhere any time soon it seems. We can't say the same for the matching denim platforms that might have been worn along with them in the pages of *McCall's* back in the day. Thank heaven!

O r, better stated, *your* nude heel! For every woman alive, their unique shade of nude is, at last, available. This is a reason to rejoice, for we couldn't say the same thing forty years ago.

Some women know nude to be a creamy color with a hint of a sun-kissed glow. Others know it to be the shade of a Band-Aid, which for years has spoken to only one segment of the world's skin. Then there are the millions of women who

THE NUDE HEEL

have avoided nude or "flesh-toned" heels because they thought they didn't exist in their chocolaty skin color, when, in fact, a chocolate brown shoe would actually be *their* version of nude.

Not unlike other essential elements of a well-dressed woman's style armory that should *disappear* when worn, from a nude seamless bra and panty to a nude lip finished with gloss or a great makeup foundation that looks no different than your bare neck (hopefully), your nude heels are critical to balanced style.

Think about that dress that has many colors working harmoniously in a Pucci-inspired pattern. The nude heel will not compete at all. If you are petite and simply hoping for the look of a longer leg, enter—you guessed it—the nude heel.

And the steps to selecting the perfect pair are as simple as one, two, three.

1: FIND *YOUR* SHADE Search for your perfect shade in *natural* light. If your favorite shoe salon only offers retail fluorescents, kindly ask your salesperson to escort you outside so you can see how the shoe color matches your skin (without hosiery). The color should blend so seamlessly that it visually melts into your skin, making it difficult for onlookers to see where the shoe begins and your foot ends.

2: FIND A CHAMELEON STYLE Closed-toe pumps should be your first investment, for they can go from work, to weekend, to semiformal evenings, and with almost any outfit.

3: FIND ROOM IN YOUR LUGGAGE Have you ever wondered why some ladies are stuck struggling at baggage claim with multiple bags, and others breeze off the Jetway and into a car with a single bag? The nude heel. The smartest, most stylish women of the jet set know the power of a single nude heel that will complement a myriad of outfits—instead of packing three or four pairs to match everything you'll wear. Not only will you save precious suitcase space, you will save time packing and save even more time wondering what to wear for dinner.

Perfect
Partners

page 158

page 77

page 195

page 104

page 218

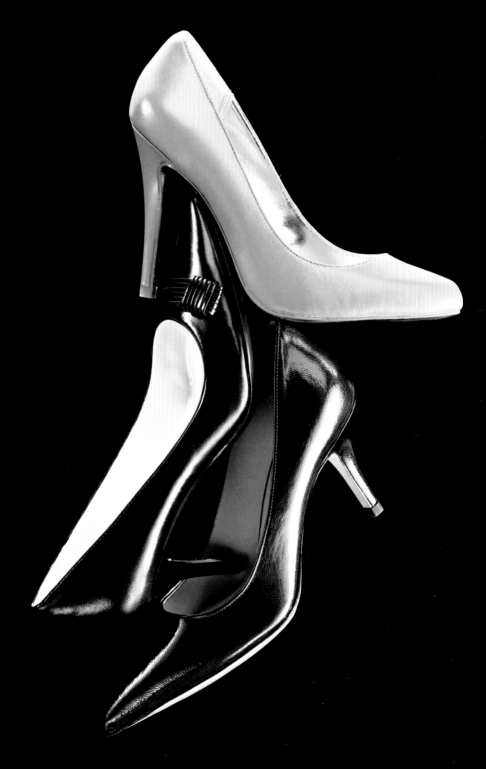

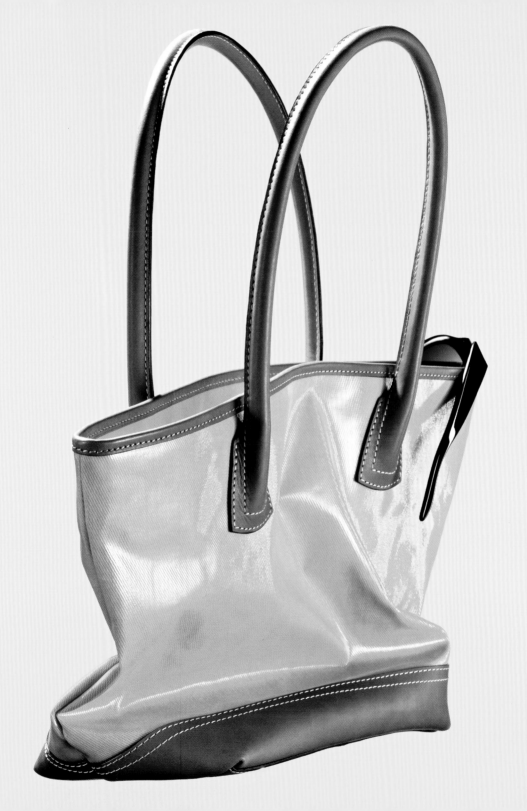

etting "dressed" to head to the water means that you want to have just enough on to be comfortable and covered and little enough to be ready to hop in and cool off at any moment. The swimsuit itself (see chapter 6) is 80 percent of the battle; the rest can be won with the accessories!

Don't settle for the proverbial giveaway tote you received at the last professional conference you attended. Leave the large handbag that you're

THE FABULOUS BEACH TOTE

trying to pass off as a beach bag at home. Leather or suede on the beach is, well, not cute.

Let the woven plastic bags spun to look like straw—with artificial daisies attached—be gone with the wind. And say good-bye to anything insulated that looks like it's meant for storing cool food.

When seeking out *your* fabulous beach tote, think of it as a big sister to your most fabulous handbag—but with a summery edge. Designers now are smart enough to offer this solution at all price points, if you take the time to look. You can find clear totes with metallic straps for next to nothing, or splurge on totes made from recycled boat sails—for a truly authentic Nantucket-meets-nautical vibe—just by Googling "bags from recycled sailboat sails."

Look out for your fabulous "designer" tote where you would shop for a great luxury handbag, or for great affordable basics, and simply make sure that the materials don't look foreign on the sand. Avoiding any animal skins is an easy way to start. Materials like neoprene (traditionally used for wet suits), organic cotton, rubberized canvas, recycled plastic, natural hemp, or fish netting top this style expert's list. These choices are fun, ageless, look right at home near sand or surf, and give a boost to even the plainest swimsuit. Embrace colors that welcome the sun, like cantaloupe, rain-slicker yellow, bleach white, peacock blue, fuchsia, and even safety orange. Leave your taste for black, navy, brown, and tan back in the "bored" room.

Perfect Partners

page 129   page 26   page 143   page 202   page 217

The wrong scarf can age you. The youthful approach to this fashion classic is achievable with the long lightweight scarf in linen, cotton, silk, viscose, or a blend of these fabrics.

Some call them spring or summer scarves; others call them wraps or shawls; I simply call them fabulous! They can quickly complete a look by adding a wink of the carefree and a nod to the wild child in all of us (even if you are corporate all week long). When you are lucky enough

THE LONG LIGHTWEIGHT SCARF

to find a version that fits your budget perfectly, is long enough to wrap around at least once or twice for drama, and is so voluminous that you feel like a star dashing from the paparazzi, buy it in as many colors as you can store and afford. Trust that you *will* wear them in warmer months, when your office dips down into igloo-like temperatures, and right through the frigid seasons for when that bulky, hand-knit scarf is simply too much once you do finally get inside. It is the perfect weight to at once balance both your body temperature and your style!

FOR WEARING WITH	YOU MIGHT CHOOSE	GO LONG/LIGHT INSTEAD
black pantsuit	black and white silk scarf	sky blue and white tie-dye
denim jacket and khakis	tan hand-knit scarf	solid tangerine
little black dress	red silk scarf	metallic silver
gray work blazer	pale blue silk scarf	lemon chiffon
navy sweater	pink printed scarf	ethnic batik print
crisp white shirt	nautical-print silk scarf	bleach white
classic blue blazer	paisley silk scarf	lime green

Perfect Partners

page 34   page 10   page 113   page 25   page 85

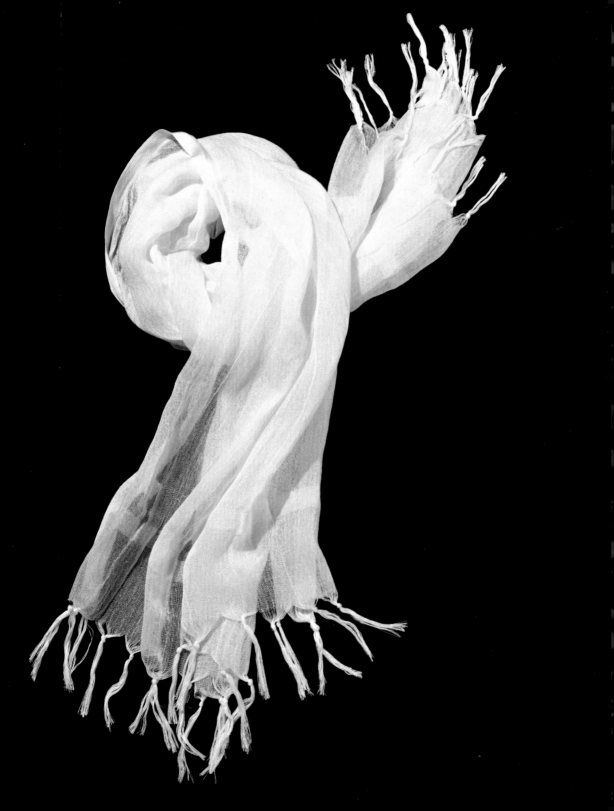

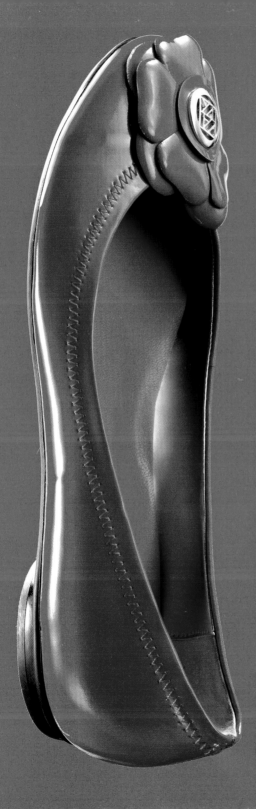

many women of a certain age wear only flat shoes. Offering them high heels is like offering a cocktail to a recovered twelve-stepper—a total no-no—and they are quick to let you know.

Younger women or the young at heart often wear high heels exclusively—and wouldn't be caught dead in flat shoes of any kind. They would rather limp home after a long day of looking tall and sexy than lose any style points by walking low to the ground with the rest of us.

THE FESTIVE FLAT

And there's nothing worse than a sad flat shoe. But there are fabulous choices to make in either category. Let's focus now on the festive flat. This is the flat shoe that looks like you *want* to wear it, not just need to because the alternative, well, frankly, hurts.

Festive flats lure the eye in with sexy shape, vivid color, bold texture, design-forward lines, and supple shine. Not only will you get a *visual* ladylike lift, but you will also look happier throughout long nights. And there's no better finishing touch on a great head-to-toe look than a happy (and comfy) woman.

Here are my top ten recommendations for styling with the festive flat:

FOR WEARING WITH	YOU MIGHT CHOOSE	TRY THIS INSTEAD
tan work suit	corporate black flats	tan-based animal print
Saturday jeans and T	trusty tan flats	buckled red patent leather
black travel pants	comfy black suede flats	silver ballet slippers
summer sundress	basic flesh-toned flats	jewel-encrusted pink flats
cocktail-hour capris	bold red flats (a stretch)	black and white zebra flats
brown church pants	reverent brown flats	pointy orange suede flats
spring shorts	basic white canvas flats	ethnic-print espadrilles
holiday ball gown skirt	matching-color satin flats	shimmery gilded slippers
comfy girls'-night-*in* jeans	run-down "house" flats	bright plaid or striped flats
date-night dark satin pants	matching dark patent flats	clear flats with a baubled toe

There are a few global style unifiers that you will instantly recognize on the backs of the most stylish women from continent to continent: A classic bold red lip, an amazingly sexy pair of black patent pumps, a crisp white shirt, and an elegant clutch bag are a few that instantly come to mind for most women. Regardless of the climate, be it a chilly night in Los Angeles, a dewy afternoon in São Paulo, or a misty morning work commute in London, if you know the essential elements of timeless global style, you will fit right in, guaranteed!

THE SHAWL WRAP SWEATER

Among the new global style classics is the shawl wrap sweater. It's usually a three-quarter-length knit creation (unless you are a true petite) that gently tops almost anything—from a tonal T-shirt and yoga pant to a button-down shirt and trousers. Think of it as a soft jacket imposter.

You might see a Frenchwoman wearing hers in black, of course, in a cashmere thin enough to silhouette her shapely figure when tied at the waist. The Italian woman jumps into it like an adult sweatshirt of sorts. It might be slightly sheer, done in white angora, and paired with a camel pencil skirt and matching knee boots.

Fly over to Rio, and the spicy Latinas along Copacabana beach simply grab it in white to layer atop their swimsuit of the day; add on a pale short-short and a metallic Havaianas flip-flop.

Your best leggings all of a sudden look more grown-up when they are shrouded by a sophisticated topper such as this—even with your best flats. The sweater you keep on the back of your office door for those chilly meetings or frigid stretches of desk work now becomes more chic than geek!

Some professional advice: Spend as much as you can on one notably luxurious version. And whether it's cashmere or cash-*miracle*, just make sure it *looks* like money.

Perfect Partners

page 122   page 9   page 103   page 107   page 214

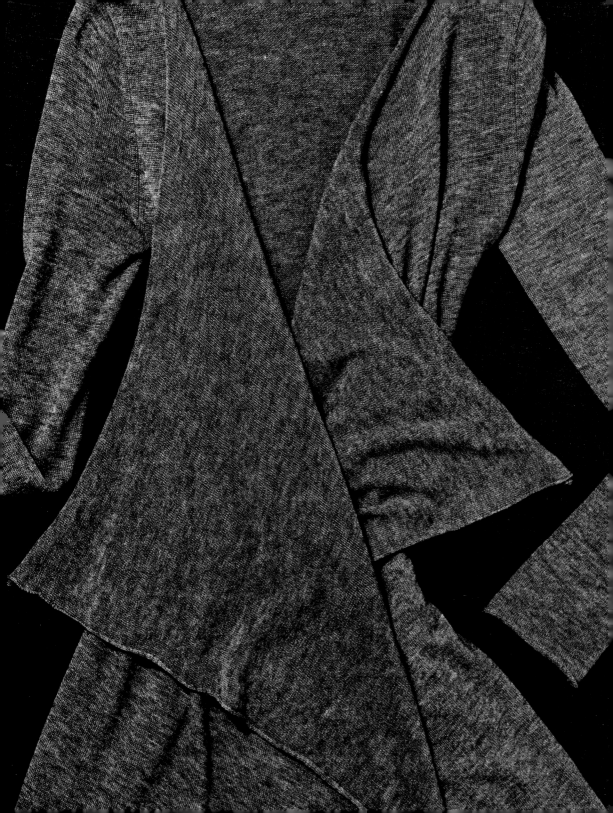

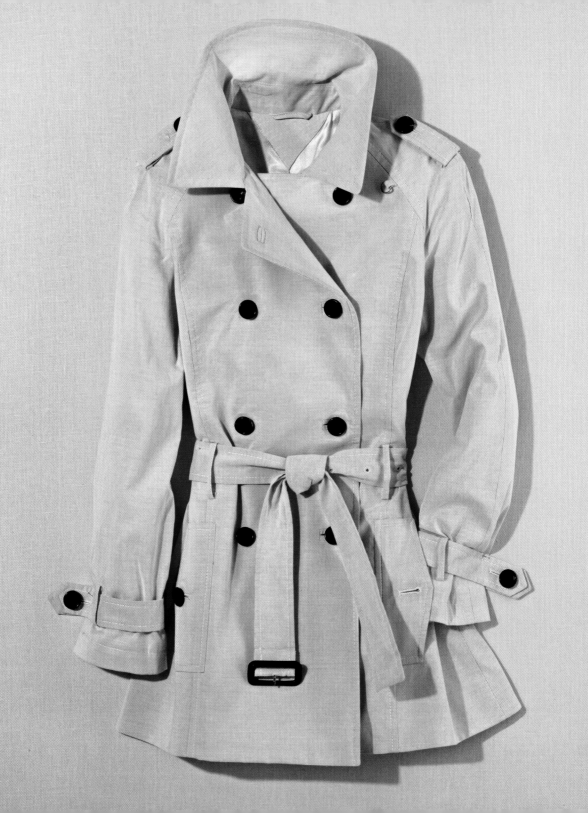

n 1914 designer Thomas Burberry was charged by the British War Office with the challenge of adapting its officer's coat to better suit the varied climate conditions of contemporary warfare. This now famous design has spawned what both men and women alike today know as the modern trench coat. The three-quarter-length tan topcoat became popular post–World War I with civilians, very similar to the way army-inspired camouflage did in contemporary times.

THE BOLD TRENCH

The permutations of the original design probably outnumber the stylish women who own them, for trenches can be found in everything from the most common thin, tan knockoff version of the original to fire-engine red nylon or even gold metallic leather—which is now offered by the originally tan-only Burberry brand. Talk about being perpetually ahead of the curve.

Ask any well-traveled woman who jaunts away often for business, pleasure, or that modernly common mix of both; her trench was most likely her first investment after repeatedly stuffing a heavy wool overcoat into tiny overhead compartments. Frustrating! And although she may now own one in black satin, a floral print, or even powder pink, she knows that you can always find another that will add even more power to your travel essentials. Kelly green might be perfect against the gray backdrop of San Francisco, while gunmetal gray is ideal for chic nights on the glimmering streets of Paris.

Keep it waterproofed (either via the hands of a professional dry cleaner or with a handy can of Scotchgard that you can mist on yourself). As for styling, belt it strong with a knot, versus using the actual clasps or buttons; pop your collar high and mysterious; and be ready to face almost any weather, having the perfect layer for almost any outfit—short of an evening gown. If your midsection looks *larger* by belting it, tie it behind you, or leave the belt at home, letting the wind create a dramatic cape effect. Either way, push up the sleeves for drama on an unexpectedly warm day, or layer it atop a cashmere sweater and wool pants for the chill of winter.

Perfect Partners

page 30   page 52   page 48   page 209   page 161

r, better yet, your flats of choice are sneakers. Sneakers for day trips out shopping. Sneakers for afternoon brunch with your girlfriends. A sneaker for that unexpected cappuccino with your better half or a new client. You can do better than that.

THE DRIVING MOCCASIN

Say hello to the driving moccasin, a flat shoe with a *slightly* active edge. Not as girly as a ballet slipper and not as rugged as your cross-trainer sneaker, this shoe gives a nod to the look of a privileged woman who drives for *pleasure*, not for purpose.

Now back to the real world, where you might be stepping out of a car full of kiddie clutter as you drop one child off at soccer and the other at a playdate. Or you are in a carpool with other women, off to spa day—finally! When you step out in your "driving mocs," you too can instantly have a look that says elegant versus plain old exhausted.

The modern genuine article is a version created in the late 1970s by designer Diego Della Valle for the Italian shoe company Tod's (formerly JP Tod's). He believed that people were in need of a well-crafted, beautiful shoe for work, play, or any elegant situation they found themselves in. He designed the Cadillac of driving mocs, which you can find to suit any part of your style—from metallic lavender lizard skin to stately black for quiet elegance.

You can find the driving shoe at almost every price point, every season—it is now a classic. This is the shoe to make you ready to leap from carpool to limo.

Perfect Partners

page 100   page 33   page 37   page 41   page 77

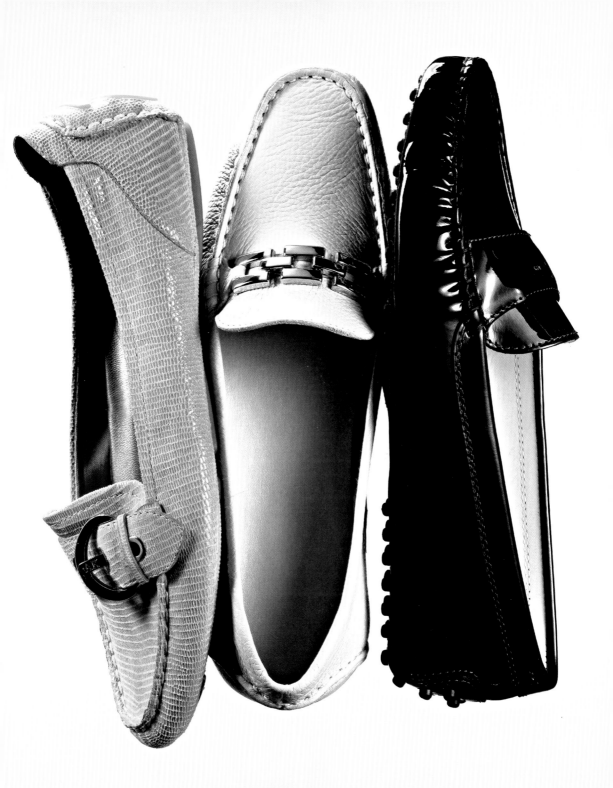

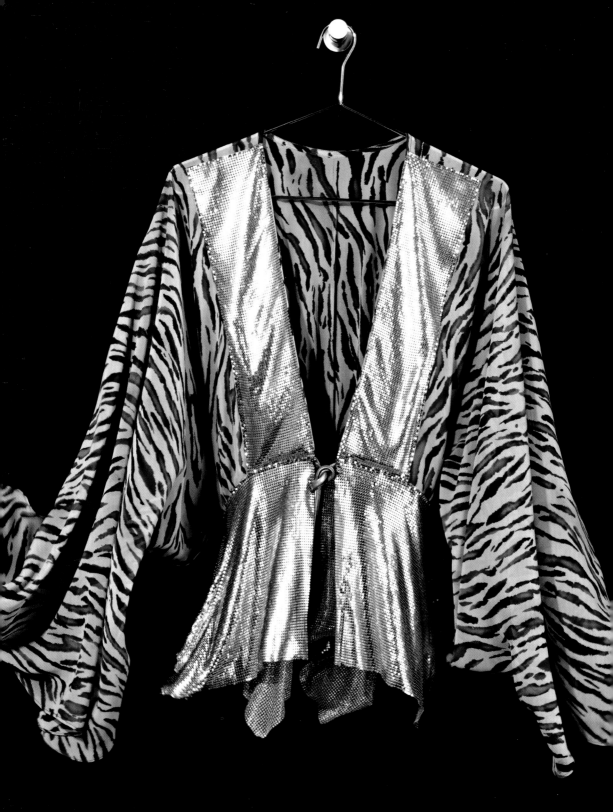

M̲ake your cover-up on the beach as modern and completely unexpected as you can. It should simply float around your body as an unexpected accent, making your swimwear appropriate for grabbing a wine spritzer on the boardwalk or running into a harbor bistro for a lobster roll. Make it a rock star item that almost stands alone and matches nothing—thus working with anything! Think leopard. Think metallic. Think shocking pink. Make it rock! Here are a few cool modern beach cover-ups:

THE MODERN BEACH COVER-UP

SHEER DRAWSTRING PANTS Yes, see-through! Legs are usually the last things to go. Incorporating a sheer pant adds a little mystery without taking away all your shape.

AN OVERSIZE CAFTAN My personal favorite instantly doubles as a little minidress.

AUTHENTIC ETHNIC FABRIC Ethnic. Cultural. Exotic. One option not to miss is Indian sari fabric, which is traditionally offered in so many colors, from spicy saffron and hot fuchsia to dreamy sky blue and crisp lime green—with many designs boasting breathtaking embroidery, beading, and shimmery metallic embellishments.

A FLOOR-LENGTH PEASANT SKIRT Tiers of joy! Grab the longest peasant skirt, whether cotton, linen, or cotton gauze. This option will balance larger hips and offer you the look of a bohemian evening gown in a pinch. Wear it on your hips, not your natural waist, for the coolest finish.

AN OVERSIZE WHITE LINEN SHIRT The inspiration here is jumping into your partner's shirt in the early morning, in the afterglow of an amazing sleep (or not).

GO ANIMAL ON 'EM! Sheer. Sexy. Beyond unique. And only if you dare to own the waterside where you lounge. The photo on page 86 says it all!

Perfect Partners

page 129   page 26   page 202   page 206   page 74

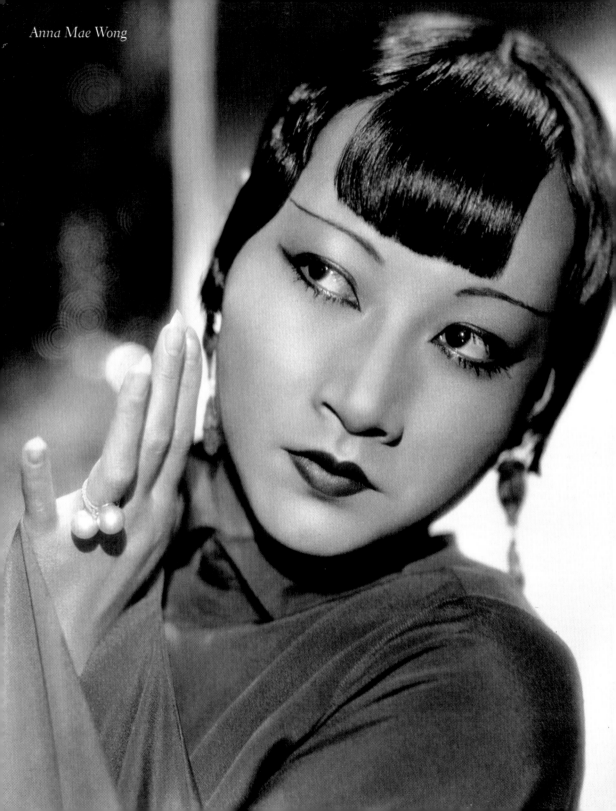
Anna Mae Wong

5 | PUNCTUATION

The fishnet stocking is most identified with the 1940s, when sexed-up "gams" were about as much as a respectable woman could reveal outside of the bedroom. The allure was the instant making of a "man trap," and fishnets haven't lost much of their appeal decades later—on the right pair of legs and styled into the best ensemble.

THE FISHNET

Something about the curved lines of the graphic design traces the shape of your stems in a steamy, alluring way that traditional hosiery could never achieve.

It can be done. The heat the fishnet can radiate can be best harnessed with bottoms or dresses that err on the side of stately, not sexy. A simple rule of thumb that you will see on the runways and red carpets time and time again is the sexier the dress, the more the fishnet should match the flesh—unless you are really headed for a consciously vampy evening.

Your black fishnets should be purchased right along with your perfect nude or flesh-toned option. And know that the smaller loops or netting offer the most sophisticated finish to any look. As you get more comfortable adding them to both night and daytime style statements, you will reach for additional pairs in a larger design scale. That's when the fun really kicks off. Just make sure you don't make a misstep by keeping a few pro styling hints in mind:

FISHNETS	PERFECT WITH YOUR	CHIC/ UNEXPECTED WITH YOUR	AVOID WITH YOUR
Black	best cocktail dress	knee boots and walking shorts	busy dresses with small prints
Monochromatic	sexiest work skirt	tweed skirt and ankle boots	job interview suits
Flesh-toned	fuller party dress	dark sheath dress	short-shorts

Perfect
Partners

page 17

page 9

page 51

page 3

page 205

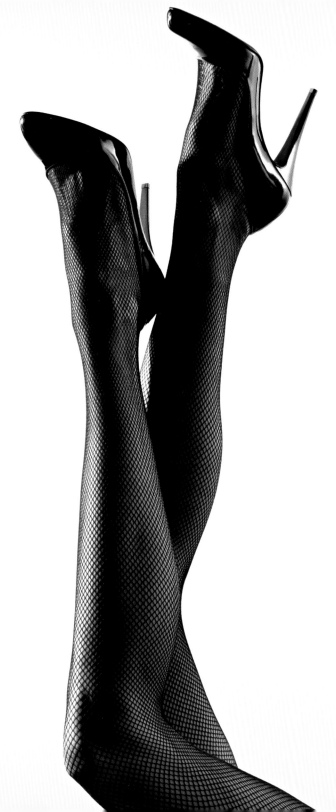

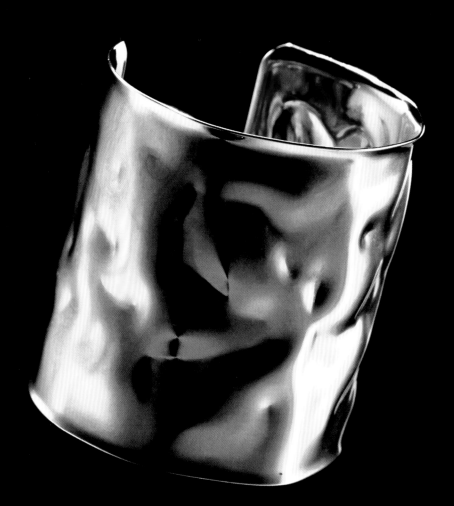

Perfect
Partners

page 60

page 56

page 187

page 103

page 202

Bold in its width, visual impact, and proportion to the arm, this finishing touch says hello, sometimes before you have a chance to. There is a built-in confidence that replaces the sweet factor of conservative sheath dresses with a hint of danger and edge. Or it can be the final detail that makes your swimsuit-and-sheer-dashiki pairing become more of an outfit than just

THE METALLIC CUFF

a haphazard cover-up and bathing suit. The metallic cuff design can be dated back to between 1000 and 1500; examples have been discovered in Incan graves with many of the basic shapes and characteristics we see today: a band of metal that tapers at each side, clearly to be worn at (or near) one's wrist.

What makes this choice stand out from the scores of other classic bracelet designs is its graphic drama and scale. For many women who choose to don one or two with a crisp tailored shirt, cuffed slightly back, it visually mimics the shirt cuff by coating the wrist with a glimmer and excitement. If you are bare armed, you suddenly have a graphic weight at the end of the arm, providing a place for the eye to rest—especially if your upper arms are not where you prefer an onlooker's eye to land.

Choosing the metal that best suits your lifestyle, wardrobe, and style signature can be the biggest challenge. A woman who keeps it seasonless and classic might opt for the Elsa Peretti design in classic eighteen-karat gold. Or maybe you are more modern in your personal style philosophy and desire a cuff that speaks to a less conspicuous touch of luxury. Then your choice should be a silver version à la Frank Gehry, an award-winning architect whose trademark lines for such artistic buildings as Spain's Guggenheim Museum have now been translated into chic metallic cuffs, both of which are evergreen mainstays at Tiffany. Only an iconic category of jewelry can welcome such unexpected artists of style and shelter to pay homage to the glory of this design.

And whether you shop at swap meets, with street vendors, at estate sales, or even on eBay, the metallic cuff will always pop onto your shopping radar. Be sure to have at least one in your jewelry lineup to add a moment of instant magic, replacing tons of wimpy "emotional" jewelry that will never visually stack up. I vote for one in gold, one in silver, and a bonus addition in copper, bronze, or pewter—just for fun. You will never again need to look deep into your jewelry box for the right *combination* of bracelets. Simply reach in, cuff it, and go!

ootwear usually offers two distinct roads to choose—high style or true comfort. And if you ask most women, the two paths rarely meet. But where they do is where the wedge heel stands. This heel design makes for a classic and comfortable shoe.

Fuller women ought to beware of the very chunky, wide wedge heels and their tendency to add more visual volume to already thick legs, and opt for a slimmer-profiled heel.

THE WEDGE HEEL

If you have slender stems though, then go ahead and try on a playfully retro thick wedge heel, if you haven't already. Most real-sized women (not runway models) have a little more flesh on the bone and need a shoe that can perfectly balance them out from the ankle region south. Choose yours carefully for maximum style impact and good proportion.

The contoured wedges you will find today are decidedly artful and playful descendants of their World War II predecessors, from clear heels fashioned of Lucite or a faux tortoise stain and matte laminated cork heels for summer to nude versions with artfully sculpted heel imprints that give a nod to the 1970s return of the wedge. Depending on the season, options will abound when you are ready to add this style staple to your repertoire.

Rotating them into your look through the seasons will offer a refreshing oasis for the foot.

SEASON	WEDGE/LOOK	WHAT THE LOOK SAYS
winter	black patent + camel pantsuit	"See me, see the CEO."
spring	linen with cork heel + shirtdress	"The early fifties just got chic."
summer	strappy with jute heel + summer shorts	"Rosie the *riveting*."
fall	colorful suede + dark denim + men's vest	"*Soul Train* sharp!"

Perfect Partners

page 152   page 206   page 205   page 34   page 217

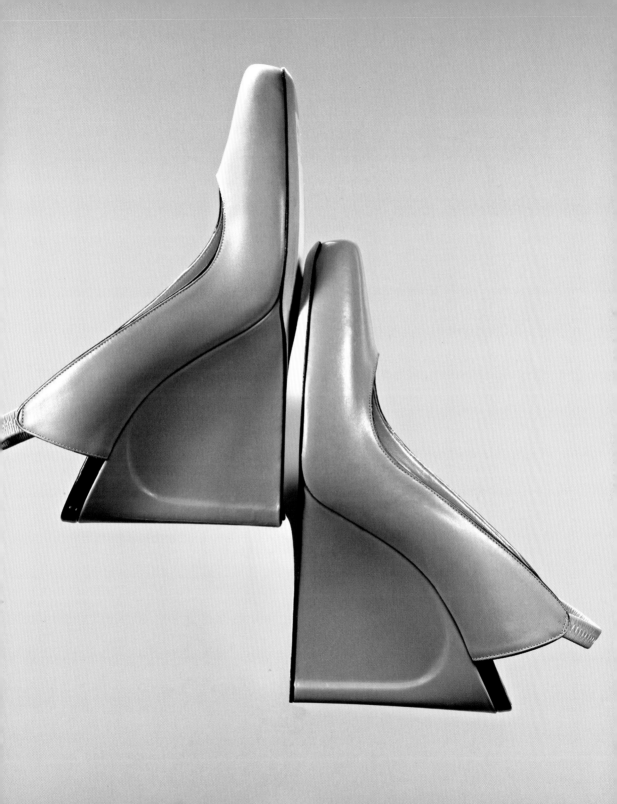

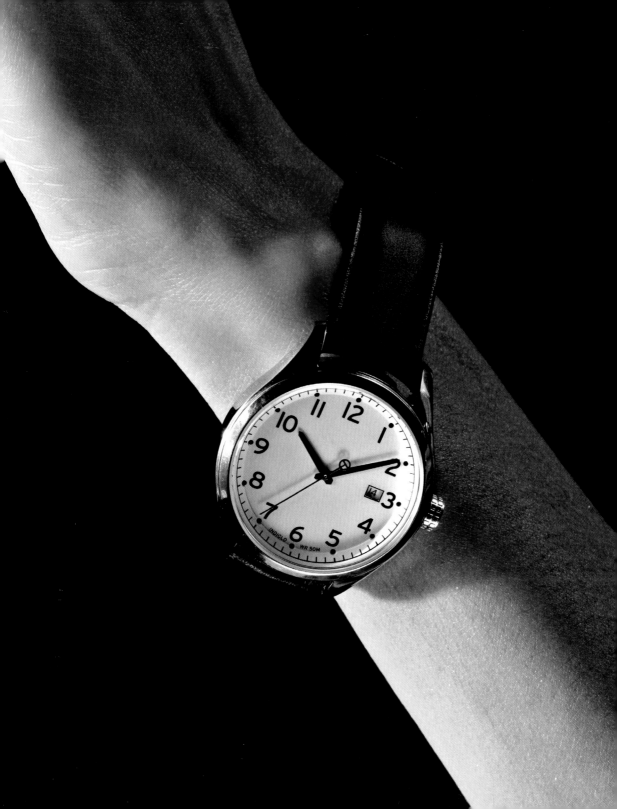

Times have changed, and *telling* time has certainly changed. When was the last time you looked down at the watch on your arm instead of referencing the time on your PDA, iPod, laptop, desktop computer, television crawl, or car clock? Accurate time is available to us every waking minute of the day, seemingly everywhere we choose to look—or not.

The art of watch wearing has suffered a great deal as technology has mushroomed

THE TIMELESS WATCH

into everything that we do and wear. Gone are the days of that elegant watch being the last thing one grabs before leaving home.

The timeless watch still has its place in your arsenal of accessories though. Wear your watch with a carefree vibe, making it almost look like an afterthought—whether it is an oversize classic Timex on a chunky menswear scale, beautifully contrasting with your slight, feminine wrist bone; a fun, youthful rubber diver watch in safety yellow by Swatch; or a thick investment piece from Panerai that glows in the night. Wear it as blithely as you would a comfy T-shirt and ballet flats. Time, shmime. Let it dangle!

A slouchy-styled watch doesn't mean that you don't know what a watch perfectly fitted to the wrist is supposed to look like—it just reads that you needn't be bound to conventional jewelry dictates and all of their airs. And just like times have changed with your clothing versus that of your mother's (is she still making sure all of her garment lengths match?), so should your spin on the accessories you choose to wear and how you choose to wear them. Loose is just cool.

Modernity is key here. Pick a watch for its character, wit, and design—not simply because it's deemed the "it" watch for its price or prestige.

Perfect Partners

page 4   page 114   page 42   page 95   page 214

paque tights are a fast and relatively inexpensive way to refresh your cool- and cold-weather clothing combinations, adding a painterly stroke of color onto even your more serious ensembles. The idea is ageless, unifying fiftysomething legs and looks right in

THE OPAQUE TIGHTS

there with what the twentyish chicks deem cool for any given season. You can give a nod to what's current simply by adding a layer of a shocking hue that revs up outfits for anywhere from the corner office to citified shopping excursions.

Get a leg up again by adding these top five motley mixed tight combinations to a newly reloaded style of your own:

FOR BUSINESS WITH A TWIST That gray skirt and cream sweater goes from acceptable to *artful* when you add opaque tights in mustard yellow. Finish off the look with black ankle boots or peep-toe pumps. Something about the partnering of gray and yellow just reads avant-garde and creative.

FOR THE ECLECTIC ENTREPRENEUR Keep a pair of deeply saturated, ink-black tights on hand to make your black wool walking shorts, black skirt, or little black dress. Add noir knee boots to finish the look.

FOR STANDING-ROOM-ONLY COCKTAILS Give your stems the edge by working a pair of tights in plum, electric blue, ruby, or even tomato—beneath a printed dress that might not have any of those colors in it! Reddish-toned tights stand on their own, especially when contrasted against cooler colors, black and white, or neutrals, just like a bold red lip holds its own with most outfits void of color.

FOR LEGS THAT RESIST The excuses abound: "My legs are too fat," "My legs are too skinny," "My knees are knocked"—you name it. Dark tights have the power to conceal and haze over many an imperfection (if you really see them as such). Many times, what you think is so obvious to others really only exists in *your* head. Black is an obvious choice, but don't forget about midnight navy blue, deep dark espresso brown, and sexy carbon gray to set you apart in a room while shrouding your challenge zones.

*Perfect
Partners*

page 196

page 17

page 202

page 161

page 187

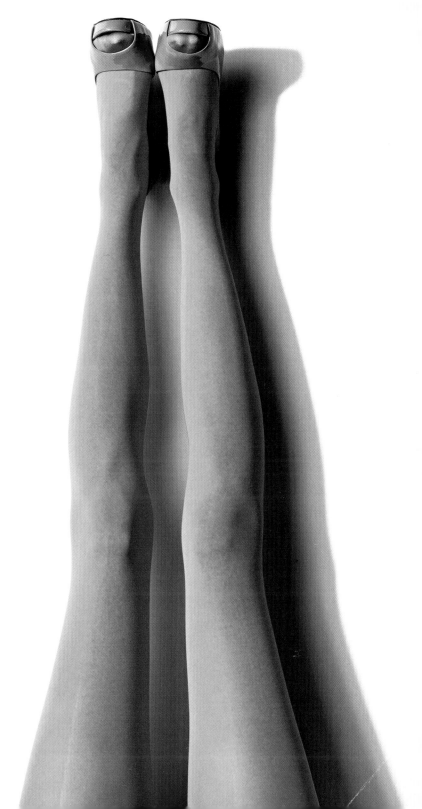

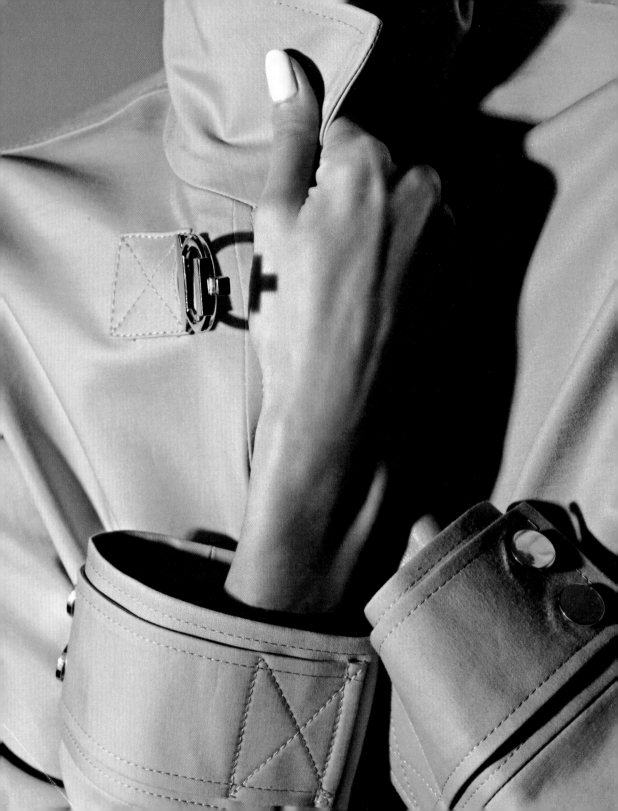

There are a few times in a woman's life when all the styling tricks and tips in the world won't be able to arm her with the confidence she'll need to look as good as she feels. Entering a room after escaping unprepared from a rainstorm is one at the top of the list.

Even your best raincoat, if chosen in tan, doesn't necessarily shine after it does its intended job to resist or repel H_2O if it is not properly treated for wet weather. And you'd be surprised how many are not treated off the rack, instantly appearing a bit

THE INCLEMENT-WEATHER ENTRANCE-MAKER

soggy and lifeless while at work, making for less of an entrance and more of a forgettable appearance at best.

Fabric technology today offers so many ways for a beautiful woman to stay that way, making your look weatherproof, rain or shine. It is amazing how many women still fight Mother Nature, with cheap raincoats and inverted three-dollar umbrellas to foldable plastic rain caps or the clumsy, last-minute folded daily newspaper—you know who you are, and sadly, so does the outside world.

Here's a tip: Look for buzzwords like Thermolite, which is insulation for warmth and is usually paired with a nylon shell. Many Thermolite coats are laminated with AquaCheck, a waterproof and breathable matte coating that protects you on unpredictable days.

Ramping up your rainwear might not top your list of style shopping tasks, unless you call Seattle or London home. I find that it always seems to be the last thing women shop for. But consider: before you opt to purchase yet another pair of shoes, trendy skirt, or designer eye shadow, upgrade your rainwear instead to save the look of the many shoes, skirts, and eye colors you already own.

Perfect Partners

page 103

page 56

page 29

page 64

page 209

What single item of punctuation separates the women from the girls when it is time to get fashion fierce? The knee boot, hands down!

Some choose to pop them on in deep chocolate brown with a classic Diane von Furstenberg printed wrap dress, where you just see a hint of skin between the top of the boot and the hem of that timeless, clingy matte jersey dress. Younger women of style smooth their

THE KNEE BOOT

sexiest dark jean of the moment seamlessly into their black boot of choice, creating the look of a long, inky leg—not unlike any fashion model or sketch. And let's not overlook the woman of a certain age who has been rocking her knee boots since the first time around in the mod 1960s. She's the gal who doesn't mind repeating a former trend that has now become a style classic—just like her. She may choose a lower kitten heel, or even a flat equestrian-inspired riding boot hybrid, but she has all the sass of the women half her age when she dons her cognac brown stunners confidently with a cream wrap skirt, matching cream blazer, and pumpkin turtleneck. She knows her body's best assets and how to highlight them, all while playing down the rest. And her boots are the strong foundation that she calls home from autumn to early spring.

Be warned, many women experience fit issues when purchasing knee boots; the designs can leave too much or too little room for the calves and/or the instep, for example. Purchase the best-quality boot your money can buy. For some women, the budget may be $200. Others may have no worries about dropping $800! Just know that the more you spend, the higher the quality *should* be, and the easier you'll slip into them. And for what fit-ease doesn't come included in the boot, a good shoe repair shop can usually provide the stretch, mending, or adjustment. Get to know your local shoe repair outpost.

But be aware that customizing a $50 boot to the tune of $75 in initial repair fees should instantly tell you that you must simply return the boot and hold off until you can afford a better version, one hopefully requiring less fixing.

Perfect Partners

page 172   page 13   page 59   page 201   page 210

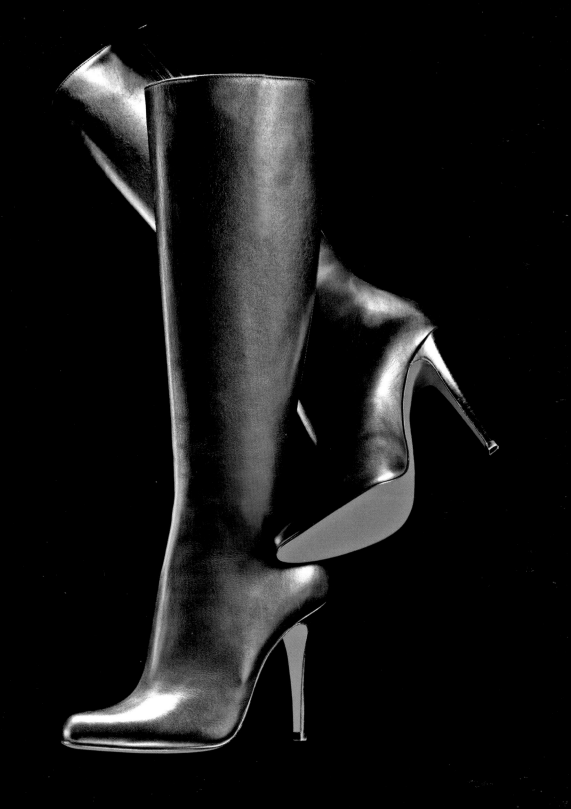

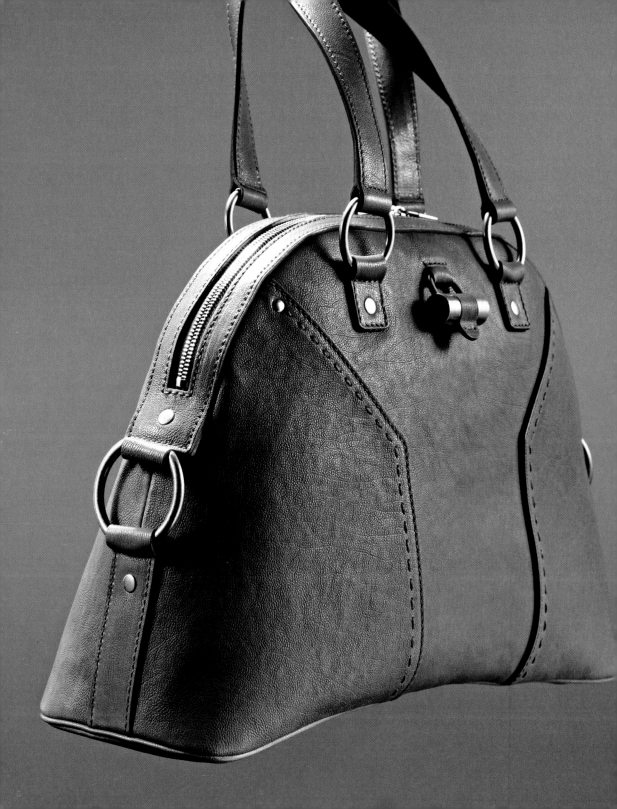

W
hen you change or freshen your look, you can instantly change or freshen your life. Instead of a potentially expensive head-to-toe revamp, I say start with upgrading something as simple as the work tote to give a boost to you and your entire outfit each day.

Here are the top three reasons to embrace the work tote.

THE KILLER WORK TOTE

3: YOUR VALUE IS VISUAL TOO Whether you step into your cubicle each business day or into the office of a potential customer, make sure that your work tote means business and style. Banish the urge to repurpose weekend totes, giveaway bags, or even worse, that graduation gift from decades ago as today's work tote.

2: THE PAST IS YOUR STYLISH FUTURE Stylists know that the best bags to be seen at eye level are sometimes vintage. Retro work totes can be quirky instead of costly. Hunt for unique and classic details such as candy-colored patent leather from the seventies, status-label prints and patterns from the eighties (think Gucci), or even a fun 1950s woven straw bag. These treatments can be costly when purchased new and lack the character of the originals. Use a small portion of the money you save to have a shoe repair shop update zippers, snaps, and metal feet.

1: GOING FROM DESK TO DINNER WILL ACTUALLY BE FUN AGAIN! Have you ever tried to dash home after work to change for an evening event ahead? Not fun. Just walking out the door begins the mad dash, not to mention the traffic getting to and fro. Investing in the killer work tote will be the answer again and again, for you can slip that slip dress, those strappy heels, that slinky evening wrap, and that sexy fragrance right inside—and maybe even a travel steamer and makeup. Your office now becomes a fitting room that saves you time, travel, and stress.

Perfect Partners

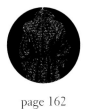 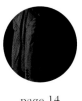 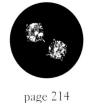

page 162   page 14   page 206   page 214   page 3

The skinny belt has been a mainstay in the closets of well-heeled, well-turned-out women dating back to its heyday in the 1940s. Picture Joan Crawford, who is one of the most identifiable screen-cum-fashion icons who did it best—especially over a strong skirt suit. Her benefit was the look of an exaggeratedly tiny waist, as compared to her legendarily pronounced shoulder padding.

THE SKINNY BELT

Today, fashionable women covet the same waist-slimming benefits this accessory provides, whether you have a super-skinny waist or not. The trick is placing the belt on the *smallest* point of your middle (which may not be your natural waist) and knowing all along that it is for fashion, not necessarily function.

Take a look at five beyond-simple ways you can grab style and benefits from a single skinny belt, for you really need only one to create a multitude of solutions.

FOR BUSINESS TRAVEL If you have a great lightweight trench, you also have a potential entrance-maker! Take out the "self-belt" that came with your trench and cinch your coat with a contrasting skinny belt instead.

WORRIED ABOUT YOUR WAISTLINE? Not sure that you even have one anymore? Or think that by adding a belt, you will only highlight an area that brings anxiety? The solution is layering the belt *beneath* a dark, slimming jacket, so that we only get a peek at it when the jacket is unbuttoned as it visually creates the look of a more defined waist. Start with a fitted or full pant or skirt; add a soft top that floats over the body (not clinging on your shape); place your skinny belt on your most flattering middle area, allowing the blouse to slightly puff and forgive; then finish the look with your jacket on *top*. If you still feel unsure, you can always remove the belt and still have a complete look.

Perfect Partners

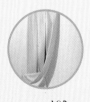

page 7   page 183   page 73   page 161   page 157

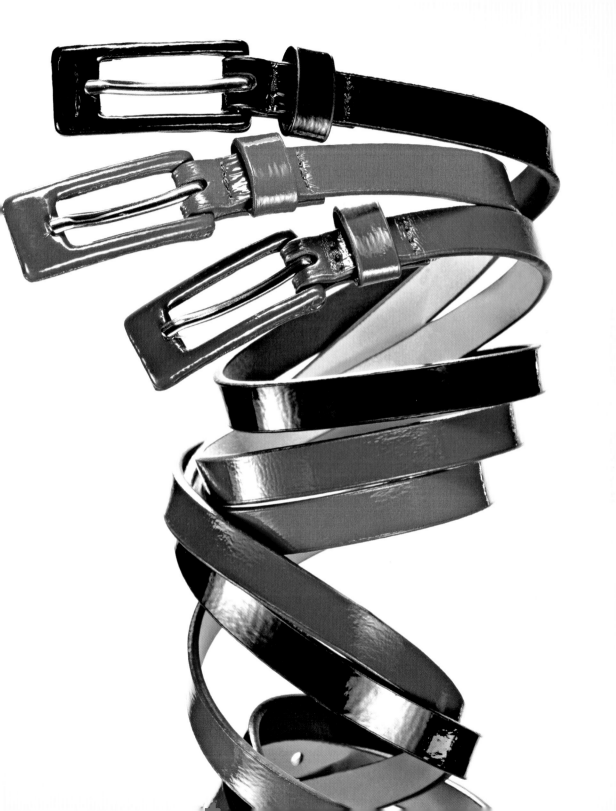

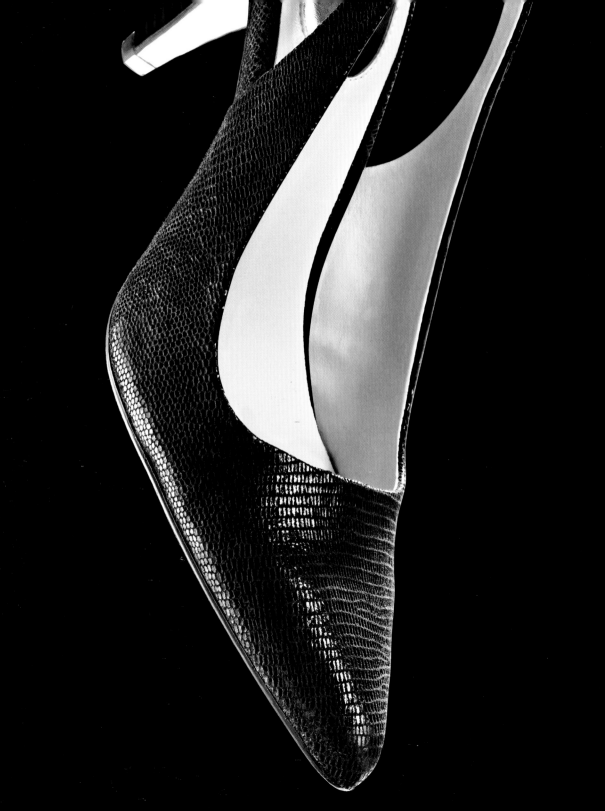

This shoe is the very definition of timeless, functionally elegant, and versatile style that garners winks and/or instant respect—the choice is yours depending on how you choose to incorporate this staple backless heel.

Slingbacks will give you universal sophistication and the ease of slipping them on and off, and they work with anything from your skinniest jeans to your smartest cocktail dress. They are punctuation at its best, for they do double and triple duty in conservative

THE SEXY SLINGBACK

workplaces and at traditional social events, and they travel abroad well when creativity and multifunctionality guide smart packing.

Keep the lines simple, and keep the material timeless; they will keep you perpetually chic from the ground up.

Perfect Partners

page 158

page 92

page 214

page 191

page 217

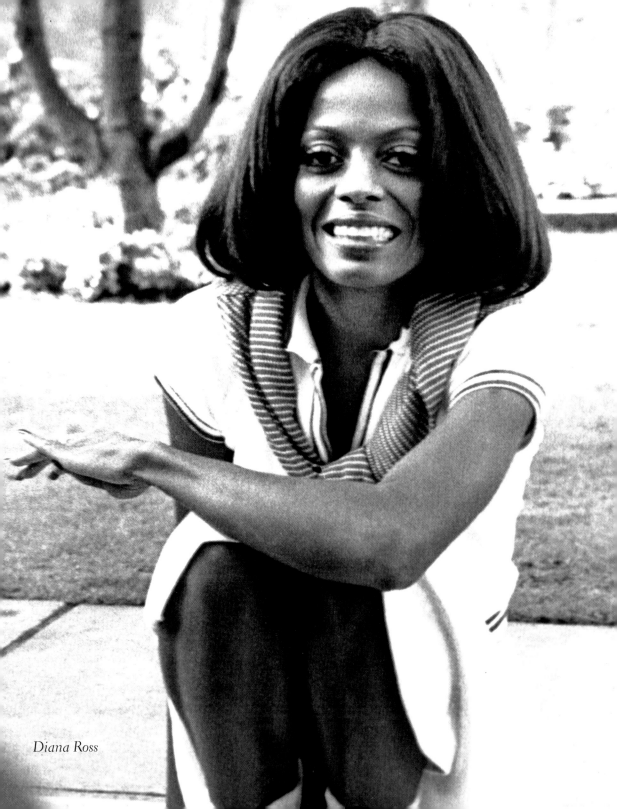

Diana Ross

6 | ACTIVE (OR NOT)

The nautical boatneck draws its inspiration from the look of the men (and women) at bustling seaport towns in the early 1900s. Coco Chanel was inspired by this now legendary classic in the seaside town of Deauville, France, in 1913, when she shockingly encouraged women to ditch the restraining corseting of the day to be comfortable. She began offering loose, liberating menswear-inspired shapes and designs such as boatneck tops, easy sweater dresses, and loose frocks accented with regimented ribbons, bibs, and authentic naval details. Chanel inspired women to dress for themselves, not their men.

THE NAUTICAL BOATNECK

And although many dismissed the idea, shunning the look as too masculine or avant-garde, the tradition of the nautical-inspired theme for *her* launched the house of Chanel the world knows today. The nautical look has been added to the style vocabularies of many of the world's top designers, including Ralph Lauren, Giorgio Armani, Dolce & Gabbana, and Michael Kors, and brands such as Jones New York, Gap, J. Crew, and Old Navy—an entire brand originally built on this very theme.

There is a breezy elegance to this style staple that sets us free. It's the perfect first mate for your easy jeans or chinos and fun flat shoes, or pop it on beneath a belted, unbuttoned white shirt and Bermuda short with wedge heels. Make it your easy and active go-to top, as the fashion world has done—and by the looks of things, always will.

Perfect Partners

page 25   page 78   page 74   page 202   page 3

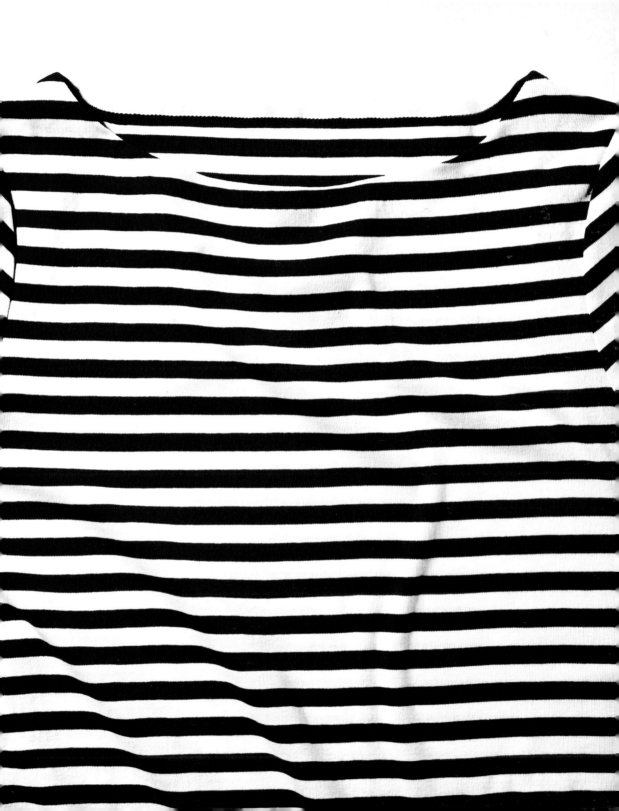

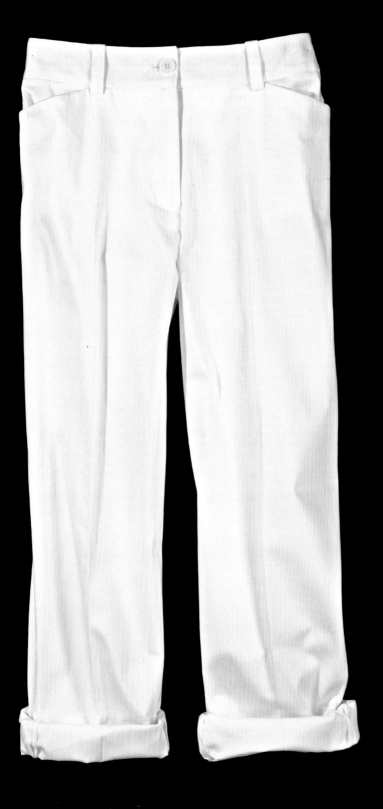

*Perfect
Partners*

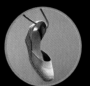

page 140

page 143

page 206

page 217

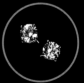

page 214

One clean easy addition to any woman's living style vernacular (or closet, to put it simply) is the capri pant. Although it originated in Europe in the 1940s from designers such as the Prussian-born Sonja de Lennart and Emilio Pucci (on the isle of Capri as Italian resort wear), many see this abbreviated trouser style as a classic *American* sportswear silhouette that is ageless, suits a myriad of shapes and sizes, and makes a strong return not just season upon season but decade after decade.

THE CAPRI PANT

This bottom had its universal heyday in the late 1950s and early 1960s as women began to finally feel confident in leaving the more traditional skirts of the early 1950s behind and empowered *each other* in choosing to be as free and easy as the men around them—but with a cropped leg hem, the signature feminine touch. Cropped pants popped up in films, television, and on the world stage like *they* were the new starlet on the scene—and the look caught fire! Mary Tyler Moore made them famous and more than acceptable every week on *The Dick Van Dyke Show.* Jackie Kennedy was the first first lady to wear them in the White House, solidifying her influence on the ease of American women's daywear. And let us not forget Hollywood starlet Dorothy Dandridge, posing for *Life* magazine in her sexy, fitted black version and keeping the heat of *Carmen Jones* ablaze in print.

Zipping to now, women know capris to be the cool, casual pants famous the world over for their feminine-meets-functional fit. You can roll cotton capris and stroll along the beach near the surf's edge or find sexy, dressy versions in silk that hug your legs and direct the eye to dangerously high heels. From stroller mom to strong creative entrepreneur, this classic idea isn't going anywhere any time soon.

Before you jump into your capris, keep in mind this style expert's top five tips:

Flat fronts are better than pleats

Petites should crop just above the ankle or just below the knee

Fuller-hipped sisters should run from tapered-leg versions (they will only add volume around that area)

Don't try them at work unless your female boss does (or male boss if you work in fashion)

Snug capris should still give you room to breathe. Don't try to pass off cropped tights for capri pants.

The quilted jacket or vest is an ideal example of something that instantly remedies cool-weather excursion conundrums that might come your way—from something as chic as a film festival in a legendary ski town to a cool crisp autumnal wine country sojourn in the Hamptons. This piece is a must!

THE QUILTED JACKET OR VEST

No more showing up for active, outdoor jaunts looking like you got on the wrong jitney, wearing a jacket or coat clearly meant for the city (you've seen *that* woman). Investing in the quilted jacket or vest the right way will allow you to mix your city style into your country day without skipping a beat—and still remain chic. Take a look at these style-forward ways to don either.

ON COLOR Choose a very lightweight quilted vest. Yes, loden green and navy blue will be standing front and center on your rack, and they are ideal investments—very slimming too. Once you own a more somber color like these, take a chance on one in butter yellow, safety orange, or grass green, even. The brighter versions will wake up dark jeans like a stylist dressed you. You can even add funk to your top half, opting for two layered boatneck T-shirts (short over long) in contrasting colors instead of the expected dark turtleneck.

ON FABRIC Select a quilted jacket in leather or suede. Take notice of a sculpted or contoured fit so you don't look like you are wearing *his* hunting jacket. This jacket looks beyond chic when paired with fitted corduroys (or tights) and knee or ankle boots. Tuck your pants in if your legs are lean; let them hang out (or cuff them up high) if your legs are on the thicker side. Either way, the jacket will welcome sensible tops (V-neck sweaters), warm tops (cashmere turtlenecks), or over-the-top tops (ruffled blouses). This jacket allows an American woman's style to swing from stately English riding influences to a sporty take on an easy Sunday without skipping a beat.

Perfect Partners

page 21   page 103   page 56   page 33   page 202

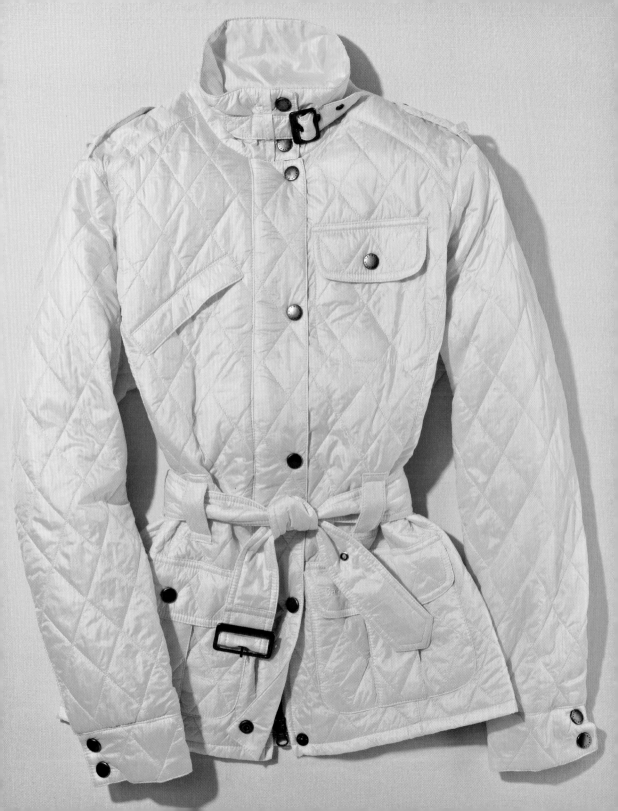

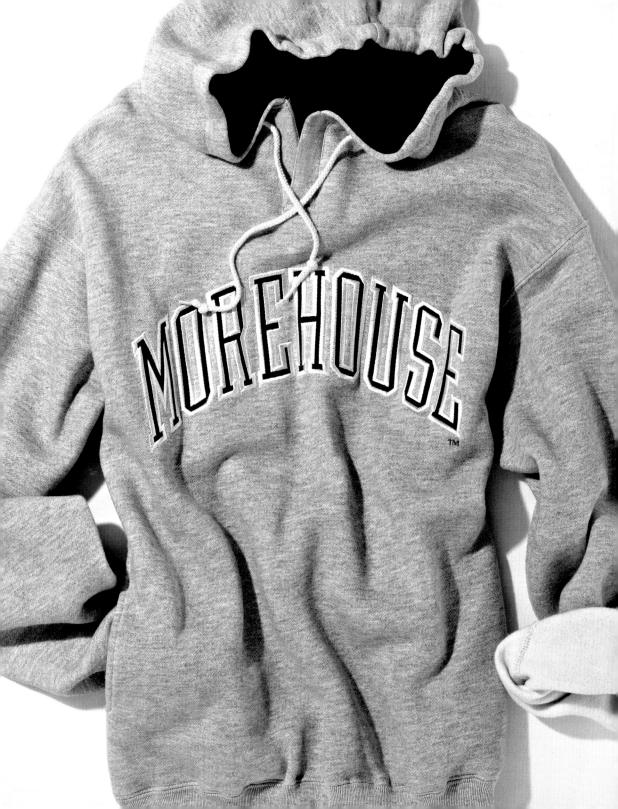

This style checklist would not be complete without the loose, slightly oversize, roomy cotton sweatshirt. This is for your days off from trying to look überchic, when you need a roomy item to allow you feel safe and cocooned. It was originally designed as a men's activewear essential. Jocks have long known the power of a chunky cotton sweatshirt, whether warming up for a game or rebalancing one's body temperature afterward in inclement weather.

THE BOYFRIEND SWEATSHIRT

Fuller tops usually look best with relatively slimmer bottoms. So your fitted yoga pants or pencil-cut capris make for a better choice than your baggy chinos or weekend jeans. Or consider a short denim miniskirt that hugs you if you want to show a little gam as you kick about town in your roomy top.

The more rough-hewn and slightly frayed quality it acquires over time from washings will only add character to its built-in charm, so let it weather—and embrace it. For you don't want to look like you went out and *bought* the boyfriend sweatshirt, but more like your mate left it at your place after a perfect night together, and you can still feel a hint of body heat and a whisper of a scent that can still make you smile.

Once you know it is yours to keep, don't be afraid to trick it out by cutting out the neckline for a nod to the 1980s. This will allow it to fall differently and open up to feature a hint of décolletage. And cutting off elastic ribbed cuffs can slightly flare the sleeve to allow a more feminine wristbone and bracelet to shine through. But don't overdo your tweaks. Keep the essence of the masculine-meets-feminine vibe for maximum style impact.

Perfect Partners

page 26

page 56

page 74

page 214

page 171

Somehow things that you might have gotten teased about during your adolescence start to become things that you now find cool. The retro sneaker might be one of them. From original Converse or PF Flyers to Pro-Keds, Tretorns, and Adidas, the sneaks that were never cool enough back in the day instantly make you feel cool and comfortable now.

This was one area where boys and girls really sported many of the same styles, so you

THE RETRO SNEAKER

might find it challenging to make today's versions reflect your womanly style. Not to worry. Forcing them into a feminine look isn't totally necessary, for the contrast can be sexy—so you have options. Here is a remix of ten ways to rock retro sneakers without missing a step.

Favorite Retro Sneaker

+ **white jeans and bright ribbon belt**

+ **white T-shirt or tank**

+ **navy blue blazer**

= *FRESH PREP*

Favorite Retro Sneaker

+ **tan capri pants**

+ **white turtleneck**

+ **newsboy cap**

= *UPTOWN, BABY!*

Favorite Retro Sneaker

+ **corduroys in color (pumpkin, corn, kelly green)**

+ **a tailored blazer in tan**

+ **a white T-shirt and a metallic clutch bag**

= *CHIC ANTIQUING*

Favorite Retro Sneaker

+ **dark-rinse denim trousers**

+ **menswear striped button-down (untucked, collar up)**

+ **stack of bangles**

= *THE RETRO ROAD TRIP*

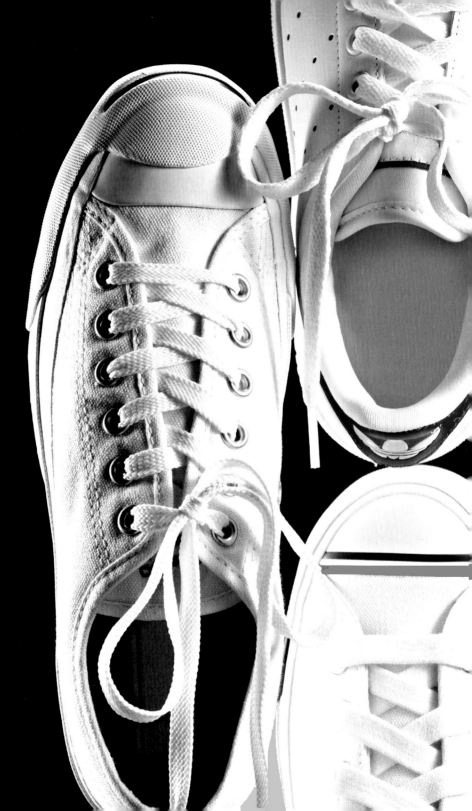

Perfect Partners

page 59

page 34

page 30

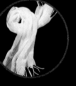

page 77

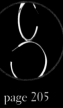

page 205

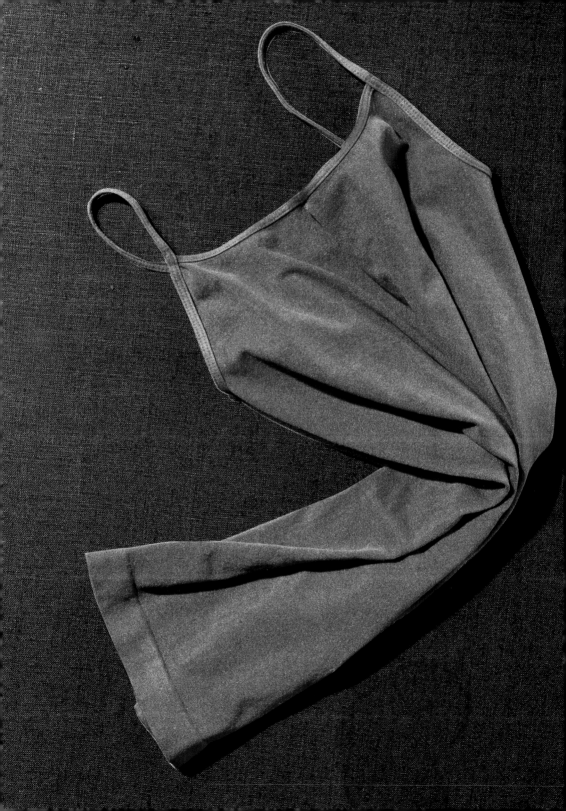

Once considered a more active, casual separate, the basic and not-so-basic tank remains a staple for women looking to relax, work out, or spend an easy weekend, but it also has the power to remix a more traditional suit, blazer, or flowing skirt. Fully embracing it starts in unexpected pairings.

You don't have to be a slender woman to feature a tank in this day and age. What you must be, though, is resourceful

THE TANK

and willing, for today's tanks are manufactured with everything from built-in bras and torso/tummy-slimming properties to a hidden double layer that actually *tapers* the waistline (with a deceiving lattice-edge hem at the bottom). Spanx makes a limited line of clothes too, with just these benefits!

A fit *look* can be achieved while you are on your way to actually *getting* fit. If you have an active look that makes you feel strong, centered, poised, and just plain sexy, it may inspire you to sweat a little more, or simply to wear clothing that no longer adds visual bulk but celebrates the frame you *do* have!

Reimagine your look with the tank in these five unforeseen pairings that will refresh almost any outfit, completely dressed up or totally cooled down.

FOR WEARING WITH	YOU MIGHT CHOOSE	TRY THIS INSTEAD
dark work suit	crisp white button-down	pink tank and pink skinny belt
business skirt	blazer and scoop-neck sweater	white tank and leather jacket
pin-striped trousers	cashmere sweater	dark tank, wide belt, and open shirt
tank dress	bare skin beneath	tank in contrasting color beneath
ball-gown skirt	wrap top or twinset	matching tank and boyfriend tux jacket

Perfect Partners

page 82   page 41   page 10   page 85   page 157

et's face it, ladies, many American women live in sneakers—and many of those same women never exercise in them. Maybe you are pushing a stroller most of the day, caring for an aging parent, or simply working in an industry where high heels make no sense at all. Those tasks are taxing enough, very much like exercise in their own right.

If you do, in fact, live in athletic footwear, at least make it artful. Not the neon-paint-spattered Keds of the 1980s

THE ARTFUL SNEAKER

artful, but artful as in a cleverly crafted design offering the look of sculpture, or an organically shaped, sleek design like that of an aerodynamically advanced car even. The artful sneaker should look just as design-rich on your feet.

The reason the artful sneaker is a closet classic, right along with items as elegant as your ladylike evening-coat or diamond stud, is the simple fact that, unlike decades ago, in today's "anything goes" society, you could actually wear them all together if push came to shove—and most people wouldn't think twice. And for most busy women, this happens more often than they would ever predict. So having all the right pieces on standby is a must.

There is clearly a way to be comfortable *and* look chic. Taking it from the ground up, The artful sneaker can set the tone for your entire look when paired with your best casual pants and a comfy, loose cotton top—especially if they are all in the same color. Going monochromatic can make even sneakers and jeans look a little more appropriate.

The artful sneaker is a wise, casual investment that won't seem as important as many of your other dressy closet classics, but it will certainly be in heavy rotation if you live in your sneaks. The trick is getting rid of the well-worn sneakers the moment your new, *designed* pair enters your world. It may be difficult, but it's totally worth the style points, comfort, and compliments that lie on the road ahead.

Perfect Partners

page 38   page 202   page 122   page 217   page 214

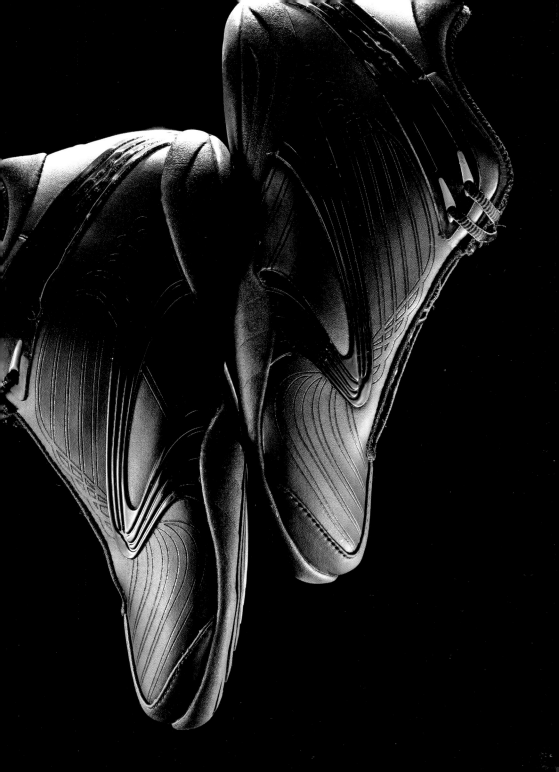

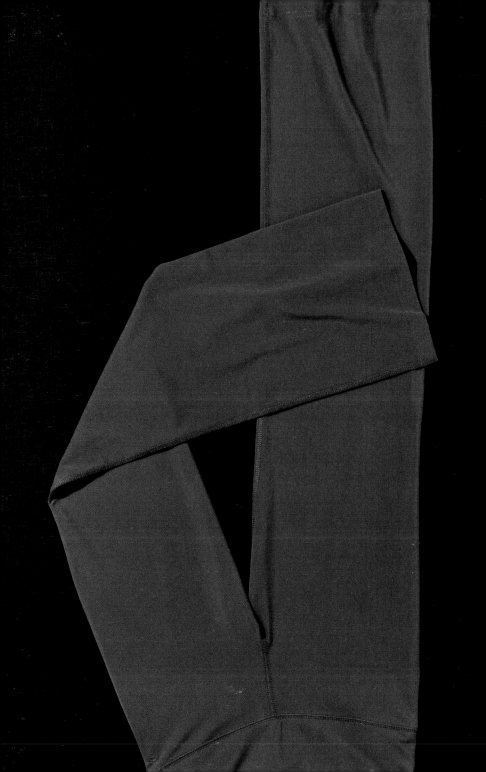

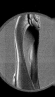

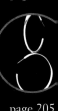
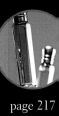

Yoga has been around for thousands of years, offering the benefits of increasing your flexibility and strength, soothing your mind, and boosting your overall energy. Many use yoga as a proven method of lowering the blood pressure too.

Conversely, what can raise this style expert's blood pressure is a pair of yoga pants that make you look more like you've been chopping and carrying wood for months. Why? Because once you know what to look for in a good-quality yoga pant, there is really no excuse not to own at least one pair that you can

THE YOGA PANT

actually be a yogi in and one you simply wear for comfort. You just have to know what to look for so the price won't put you into a downward dog at the register.

For women who are active yoga enthusiasts, there are rules that make your time on the mat more productive. Since your posture is critical when posing, you want to wear garments that stretch and skim the body—and not just for you, but so your teacher can actually see how your body is positioned, guiding you as you go along.

Anyone who has successfully taken even one yoga class will testify to the high sweat factor. And although from the outside it may look like you are sitting around an imaginary campfire, the only thing burning will be *you*, from the inside. Especially in Bikram yoga, which takes place in a heated studio. So, in general, your clothes should be in the latest quick-dry fabrics and have moisture-wicking properties.

The best yoga bottoms will be offered in a myriad of styles and details to suit *your* unique figure. There's high-rise (best for long-waisted women), low-rise (for their short-waisted counterparts), reversible versions that help your body and budget, ones with slim legs (for slender women), and ones with wide legs (for gals with ample stems and hips)—a yoga pant isn't just a yoga pant anymore. Many better brands even come in regular and tall lengths, and in fabrics suited for warming up or just for cooling down. So finding *your* best bottom is so worth it.

Most important, if you can invest in two pairs, start with a double dosage of black. Keep one for actual use in the gym, yoga class, or Pilates studio, and ride it till the seat wears out. Reserve the second pair to be worn only *after* your workout, so they always remain fresh and camera-ready, if you will. That's the pair you can dress up and never get a second look (for the wrong reasons). You can branch off into other colors later, once you get the hang of keeping one for sweat and one for style.

s there such a thing as the one perfect swimsuit? Better yet, is there such a thing as the perfect body? The answer to both is no. Thank heavens!

One swimsuit idea that does come close, though, is the classic maillot (mah-'yoh), the one-piece wonder that we've seen the world over since the early 1900s. The maillot doesn't have to be boring or for "old ladies" either—unless you start chasing versions with that skirt that

THE PERFECT SWIMSUIT

can make you look even fuller at the hip. If you keep it clean and understated and opt for a moderate leg height and a self-supported shelf bra (if you need it), not only can this choice be tasteful and sophisticated, it can also read as sexy and elegant, something that the girls donning their two-piece thongs can never say.

Simplicity is *critical* when looking to invest in a singular swimsuit that will soon become your best friend, as your body gets "sometimey," as they say in the 'hood. Most women know all too well how much of a fair-weather friend your figure can be.

From a style standpoint, a classic, ever-tasteful swimsuit has a neckline that offers just a hint of décolletage, fabric that just skims the skin (20 percent Lycra will help to balance out the nylon and add snap), and a deep color that shapes you to the eye (anything but black to start). This style expert votes for midnight ocean, black plum, or even a deep slate gray— colors that celebrate the sexiest palette of nature yet still have similar slimming qualities to that of basic black.

Your straps are not only what keep your suit on but also what keeps your style interesting, for they are a place to express your unique take on the season without compromising your most comfortable fit. Elegant chains, braided metallic leather with a waterproof finish, or even a self-strap with tonal embroidery can offer options for making your swimsuit a nighttime top in a pinch. So have fun with those two zones, and select a look that will not only add interest, but maybe even distract the eye, if you need that to happen.

A fully lined front and back are important, especially when featuring your suit at group events or crowded, sunny beaches—unless you are in Europe, where suits sometimes get peeled off as quickly as we here in America peel off the cap to our sunscreen—if not faster.

Take a good, *long* look in the mirror, and take a good longtime friend, when shopping for your perfect swimsuit.

Perfect
Partners

page 26

page 214

page 202

page 143

page 74

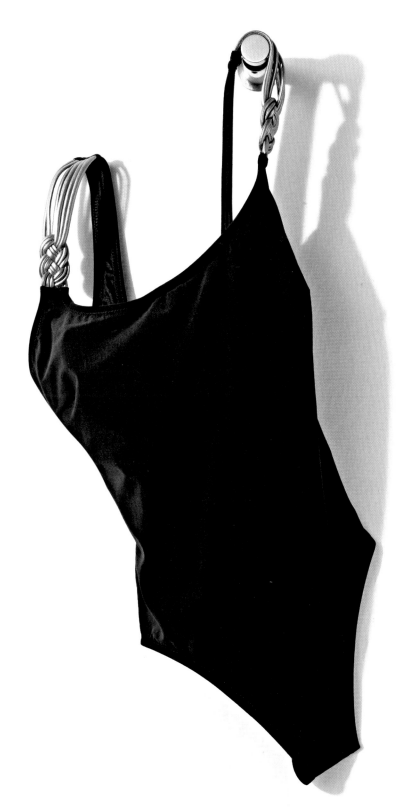

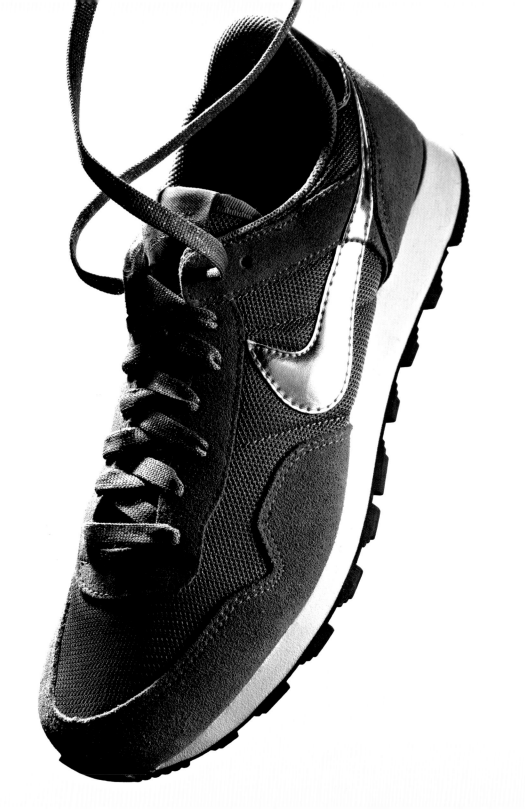

Adding a reserved cross-training sneaker to your wardrobe may sound less than stylish. And what I mean by "reserved" is simply that you reserve its use only for your workouts in the gym. You promise yourself never to wear them in a pinch for yard work, rainy-day mailbox runs, or any really rugged outdoor activity. You almost treat them like good high heels that never touch the ground during your pedestrian commute time. With this care, they will always look as good as they did new, while still providing the support you need and the style they originally boasted.

THE STEALTH CROSS-TRAINER

Usually made of leather, combined with a mix of other flexible materials, cross-trainers are an amalgam of various athletic sneaker styles, good for everything from tennis and running to aerobic dance activity and weight training. Quality versions should boast solid cushioning for your forefoot for jumping, the heel cushioning of a shoe designed specifically for running, and side support for a good game of basketball or tennis.

Although sneakers may not seem like an obvious closet classic, most women would live in casual clothes if they had the option. And cute sneakers have become a huge part of workout attire for most busy women today. With this in mind, they should be focused on a bit differently than you may have in the past. For if your "sneaks" are to be seen in the gym, a single quality pair chosen for their high style, durability, functionality, and comfort is a smart solution. Sometimes a boost of style is exactly what you need to get motivated and moving.

Perfect Partners

page 122   page 126   page 37   page 33   page 214

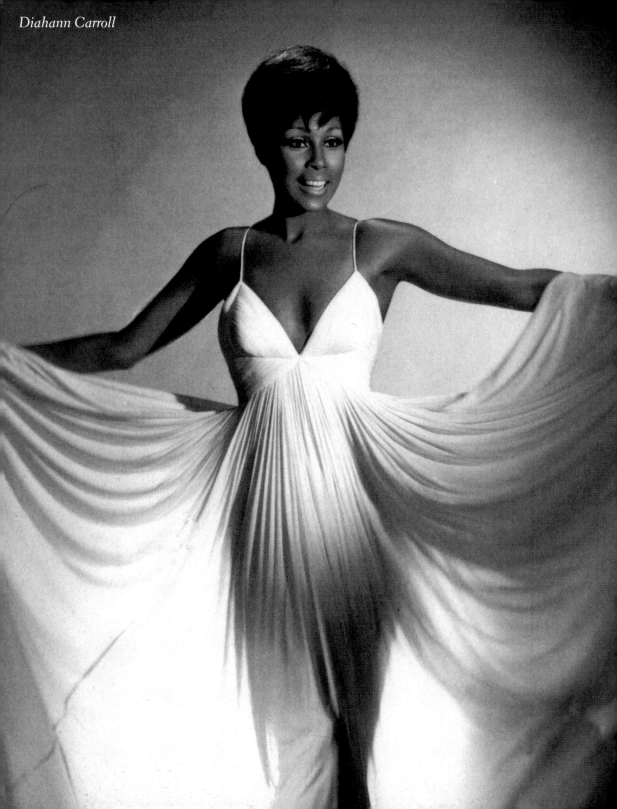

Diahann Carroll

7 | ENTERTAINING

Opening the doors to your home for any type of event is a chore unto itself. The preparation means different things to different hostesses. Some leave it all up to hired help, giving themselves loads of time to look like a star when guests arrive. Others try to do it all and reserve mere minutes to throw themselves

THE DRESSY FLAT SANDAL

together in a panic. Which are you? Have you ever taken a good long look at your style of entertaining and how your planning choice impacts your entertaining style? Know that your guests have.

A dependable way to start adding style from the ground up is the flat dressy sandal. So even if you wind up opening your door in your yoga pants and a T-shirt after a long day of prep, there is at least a festive touch that finishes your style sentence.

Integrating this moment into your footwear lineup couldn't be simpler, for the best versions of this idea are stand-alone design expressions that need not relate to or match anything else in your closet.

Think of this type of sandal as charms for the foot! And many of today's flat sandals come with crystal embellishments, exotic beaded detailing, jewel-encrusted accents, and even metallic leather crafted to resemble soft flower petals—and these ideas just skim the tip of what's out there to enhance the foot.

"Dress" might be the wrong choice of word to describe a flat sandal. But it does dress up a more casual look. Socializing and dressing—even for business—are increasingly more casual, and women are getting busier, so comfort is becoming a more important factor to them. The flat dressy sandal should have a firm footing in your shoe lineup.

Wear with your jeans and go from errands to entertaining just by adding a cute top or soft blazer. A long, tiered peasant skirt will welcome their addition for walks into town while on vacation in a swimsuit. Even that summer work suit looks great with them on your commute, and you can pack your heels in your tote—a better way to achieve comfort during your commute than sneakers or your rubber flip-flops.

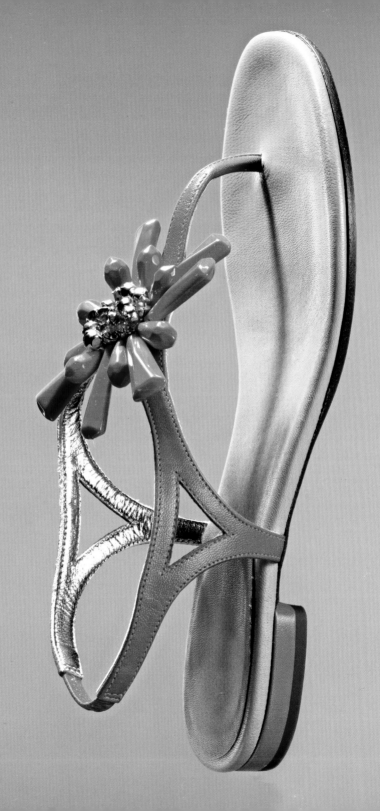

Perfect
Partners

page 143

page 147

page 202

page 166

page 217

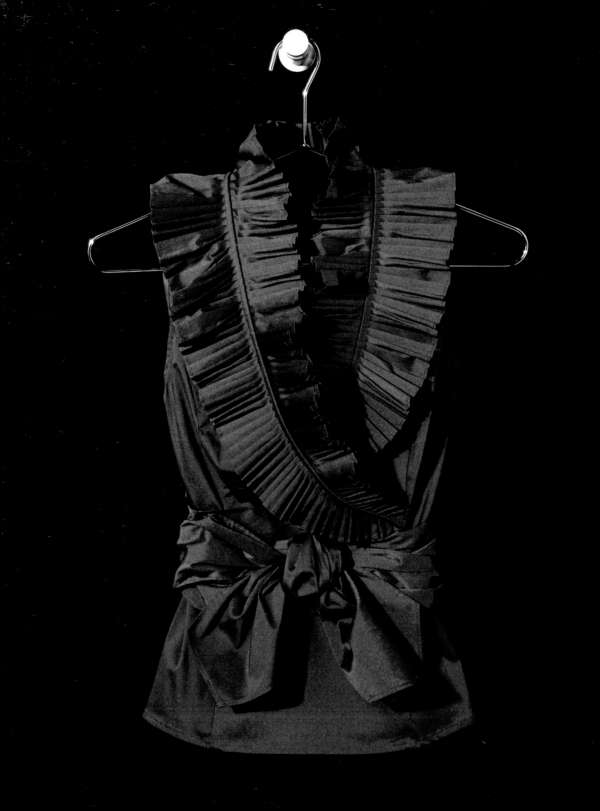

Queen Elizabeth I got it right; when greeting a room full of guests, always frame the face if you want to let them know who's really the hostess in charge! Her signature ruff, a sort of wheel-like, pleated, staunch white collar (sometimes bordered in an intricate lace) projects epically from her neckline in most of the paintings and film depictions of her to date. It was the 1500s, and showing a hint of skin was not an option, even for *the* most powerful woman in the world. Can you imagine?

THE RUFFLED TOP

The ruff design was a fore*mother* to what we simply know today as ruffles. They show up over and over again in the collections of the legendary Latin überdesigner Oscar de la Renta. The festive look also conjures up the wonderful silver-screen legend Carmen Miranda, a.k.a. "the Brazilian Bombshell," whose trademark ruffle-edged dresses gave a shocking nod to her Portuguese roots in an era when neatly tailored skirts and dresses were de rigueur for most actresses on the world stage. Not to mention her turban full of fruit!

The ruffled top, whether sleeveless, slightly low cut, or simple and smart, is as ageless. The artful drape and flow of the actual ruffle just says beauty and grace, directing the eye up to a gorgeous lip color, a dazzling smile, or a wonderful pair of earrings nestled into softly coiffed hair.

Today's versions have been reimagined and reinterpreted to make even a grandma who tries one on look chic again—especially when she rocks one with her dark-rinse denim trousers or black satin cigarette pants. As for granddaughters, and all women in between, the ruffled top looks so right when layered beneath a sharp, fitted black blazer, allowing the billows of ruffles to rise out like a soft arrangement of flowers. Add a jaunty pant or pencil skirt to complete a style that speaks to the signature looks of Yves Saint Laurent—namely his famous "Le Smoking" tuxedo suit. *Très chic!*

Perfect Partners

   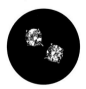

page 9   page 103   page 171   page 214   page 161

spend many days out of the year in cities across the United States, dressing real women of all ages, most of whom are not celebrities. I treat them all like stars as they artfully balance their family, home, and career. This is when and where I enter. I help make them *look* like the stars I know they are.

THE FLORAL STATEMENT PIECE

The floral statement piece can add the perfect special feminine touch. Let it share the stage with other more traditional, ladylike wardrobe essentials such as the evening sandal, the ball gown skirt, and the signature scent, just to highlight a few.

TWENTYSOMETHING Get yourself some party pants in a floral print. You may be too young to remember the floral pedal pushers for nonstop beach-blanket fun in the 1960s or the dancers who backed up the Supremes on Ed Sullivan wearing their cheeky cropped pants while doing a mean mashed potato. But know that the party pant has only gotten better with time. Versions with bright colors and metallic threading are tops!

THIRTYSOMETHING The floral dress is an easy way to make a fashion statement without looking like you are trying too hard. Here's a pro tip: Make sure no flower motifs fall on areas of your body that might be "in progress." Ask a good girlfriend to check all sides before you ring yours up.

FORTYSOMETHING All florals aren't equal. Some smaller, scattered flower designs speak to the sweeter, predictably more mature side of your personality. The larger, more graphic versions might be moving you over the hill faster then you can say "Boniva"! This is the decade to choose a more *abstract* floral. Ink-washed renderings that look hand done, Asian-inspired flora on everything from topcoats to near-sheer blouses—you have options. Your style is now *made*, as they say in the mob. So make it work beautifully for you by rethinking florals, wearing just the right dosage to spice up a look. A handbag, a long summer skirt in gauze, or just a fun layering T-shirt are easy first tries if you are hesitant.

FIFTYSOMETHING AND BEYOND Color floral prints are fine, but black and white florals reign supreme. Something about the timeless, graphic nature of this choice speaks to your ageless style while remaining sophisticated and current. Pop it with accessories and layering-piece accents in bold colors like marigold, tangerine, or even tomato. Side note: These are the *only* fake flowers that should be in your world from this decade forward.

Perfect Partners

page 59

page 205

page 34

page 217

page 161

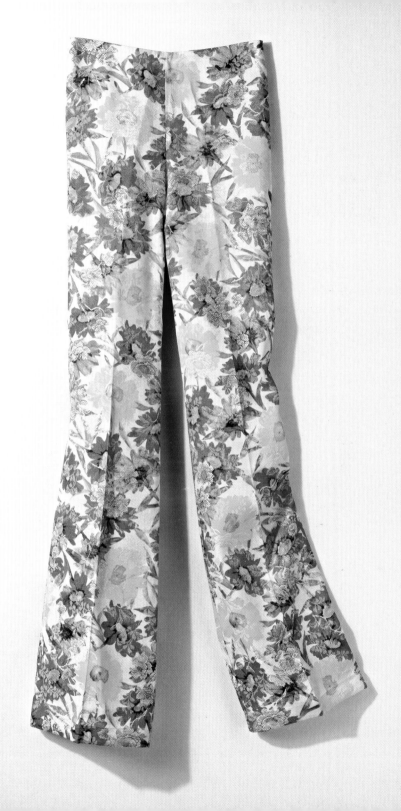

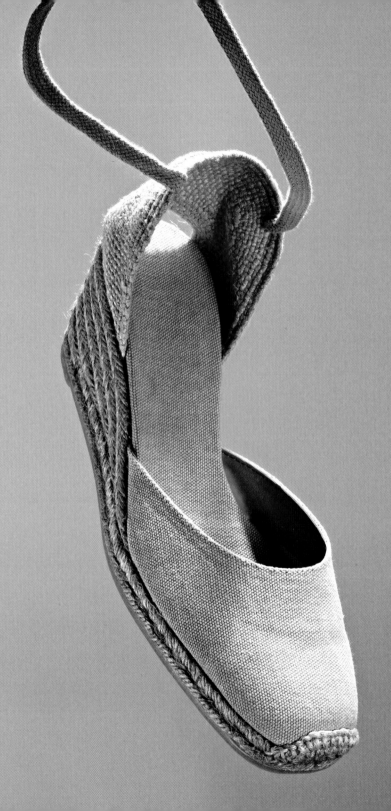

Perfect Partners

page 55

page 56

page 171

page 214

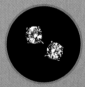

page 107

What makes an item a closet classic is usually the item's ability to stand on its own as a solo investment. That said, the espadrille, when spotted at an amazing price, is a classic flat shoe that is best purchased in an array of colors and styles.

The espadrille is a time-honored comfort solution, having been made in Spain since the fourteenth century; this simple-cum-elegant design was also "green" well before Earth was put in peril by man. With its natural jute (a plant fiber used to make rope) sole and natural woven cotton upper, the eco-friendliness

THE ESPADRILLE

factor is high, and the instant style recognition is even higher, whether they're featured in Barcelona or Brooklyn. Those who know timeless spring and summer style know the espadrille well.

When investing in your perfect version of this shoe, look for a rubberized sole to provide a thin layer of water protection. Authentic versions that don't offer this modern finish will absorb a rainy day and literally swell on your feet, making it difficult to get out of them.

As for color, this is a moment to practice a touch of reckless abandon, especially if you find a pair of espadrilles that fit snugly into your discretionary styling budget. Some summer street fairs will still offer a pair for a crisp ten- or twenty-dollar bill, a nod to their dwindling hippie following. And even style-at-a-steal stores and websites such as Target, H&M, and London's Topshop (which has finally arrived in the States) will have them available for well under what you'd pay for any leather-soled flat spring shoe.

Think fruit stand when you hit the right price and grab a pair in mango, kiwi, strawberry, plum, banana, cherry—the list goes on—not to mention fun stripes or ethnic prints and patterns like batik or ikat. This way you will have them on standby for any casually chic outfit you dream up at home or on the road, for they are also a collapsible packing dream.

Even when you're entertaining, you too can feel like a guest when you are wearing the right footwear, and the espadrille is perfect for hostesses in warmer months outdoors and even cooler months *indoors*. Pop on a crisp white pair with cropped pants and your best swimsuit for summer fêtes by the pool, or be the envy of the pinched-toed, high-heeled guest at your own winter holiday soiree when you feature a red or black pair with your favorite white jeans and a black cashmere turtleneck!

The invitation asks for guests to arrive at seven. It is six thirty, and you have just finished arranging the flowers, plating the food, chilling the bubbly, and arranging the room so that it is just so. And just as you are about to dash in to freshen up, gloss your lips, and choose an outfit, the doorbell rings. Early! For there is always that one "helpful" friend who thinks that by showing up a wee bit ahead of time, she's helping you. Wrong! All she's doing is cutting in on your glam time.

THE FAIL-SAFE HURRIED-HOSTESS TOP

The remedy is the hurried-hostess top: the tunic. Some call it a caftan. Its power is limitless for just about any party, any season, any year, for it has been stylish for centuries. Talk about timeless; it might not get any better than this festive and flattering staple that has been like the T-shirt of the Middle East since forever.

Here's how to wear your tunic for just about any occasion.

THE INTIMATE DINNER PARTY Grab the tunic that has the most festive ornamentation, from intricate neckline beading that reflects candlelight onto your face for photos, to breathtaking appliqués around the cuffs to grab the attention of all guests when refreshing drinks. Go for intense color too, fuchsia, lime green, peacock blue, or intense lemon—this means less dinner and more party! Cool it down by wearing it atop comfy dark leggings or your best yoga pants and flats with a touch of shine.

THE OUTDOOR FÊTE Ditch that staid sarong and opt for your caftan instead when it is time to host (or attend) a pool party. Or make your Bermuda shorts have shock value by coupling them with a fresh white tunic for a barbecue—when every other woman reaches for her basic sleeveless button-down summer shirt.

THE HOLIDAY ROUNDS Whether fireside or at Grandma's side, make your holiday rounds chic again by opting for a tunic instead of that chunky sweater that speaks of the season's cartoonlike motifs. Yikes! In general for this time of year, as your coat keeps you warm outside, there is usually no need for a heavy top inside. Once you peel it off, you will be the guest in the beautiful navy tunic, white cords, and cute orange flats that everyone is murmuring about.

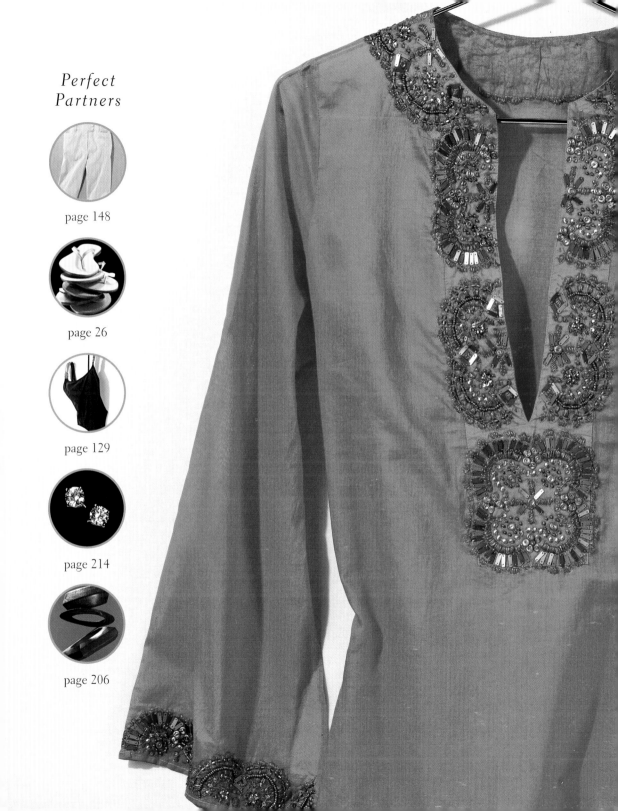

*Perfect
Partners*

page 148

page 26

page 129

page 214

page 206

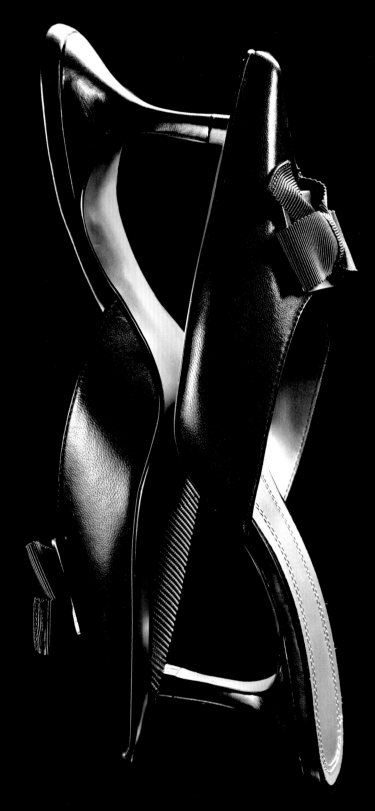

The mule, which is simply a backless shoe, usually ranging from medium heels to flats, holds a firm place in the wardrobe of classically styled women who need not rush when leaving their door. And although the shoe's practicality ranks low, its posh factor soars sky-high when it's time to finish off a look without appearing heavily styled. And animal-like nomenclature aside, this dressy slipper has an instant look of success, for its casual fit and flop speaks of woman who is anything but pedestrian or on the run. The beauty of this look is that you might

THE MUST-HAVE MULE

very well be on the grind, but something about adopting this footwear choice, at least in that moment, allows you to assume the look of the ranks of the women who *aren't*. Knowing the world's style shorthand is a powerful tool in creating your day-to-day image, so use it!

If fashion had a hall of fame, the mule would sit right next to iconic design ideas as renowned as an elegant strand of pearls, a simple white T-shirt, or an evening glove—all of which can be worn high *or* low these days. You'll see it on the red carpet one moment and in a cool downtown pub the next. The mule will shift between settings as easily as your best tailored separates when you know how to make it stand out or fall back.

So when *is* the mule the ideal choice? The answer is short and simple: When you need to send a message and let a room know that getting dressed, for you, is more of an artistic ritual and less of a hurried necessity. And we have all seen how that can look.

Juxtapose the power of this lazy-cum-luxurious heel or flat with a more serious outfit. That pantsuit that gives a nod to menswear but seems to look a little too manly when worn with thick-heeled pumps, even. Something about a smidge of skin peeking out of the back of your shoe, atop a slim heel, instantly ups the feminine quotient in even the boxiest of menswear-inspired garments.

A big no-no: hosiery with your mules, unless the hose are the footless kind. Otherwise you'll be sliding into home base—and not in a good way!

Pants with a slight crop to them, just grazing the bottom of the ankle, will allow the mule to get its deserved spotlight. Capri pants are even better. As for skirts, they look the strongest with versions that split the knee, whereas longer skirts tend to steal away a bit of the wearer's youth when paired with mules. Something about the length of the skirt or dress paired with the slipper is reminiscent of an older generation, so unless that is your goal, they are served best on the sassy side.

The linen pant should be the first thing on your warm-weather entertaining checklist.

Let's talk function first. Many women immediately run to their cotton clothes for hot outdoor events, thinking they will remain the coolest. They avoid linen garments for the wrinkling factor. This thinking should be reversed.

THE LINEN PANT

One hundred percent linen fabrics in most weights and qualities are actually *more* absorbent, stronger, and cooler than your go-to cottons. And, if you look, many of today's linen garments are treated to resist wrinkles as you go about your day in the sun.

When looking to incorporate the linen pant into your fashion vocabulary, be certain to keep these three key points in mind.

GO NATURAL From pure optic white and ivory to warmer earth tones like flax, tan, toast, sand, cement, and even pale caramel, what's really in a color name? Just know that your first pair should be pale and warm. This choice will give you the option to toss just about anything on as a top, from a casual and bright persimmon tank to a chic cotton jacket in nautical navy blue. And don't worry about your lower half looking thicker due to the pale color. The linen pant is meant to float around the leg, offering ease and forgiveness, no matter your size, so size it up if necessary.

STRING YOURSELF ALONG Drawstring-style linen pants are first cousins to your tried-and-true favorite pajama pant style. Look for full stovepipe legs, optional pockets, and a self-belt built into the waist as a slim drawstring. No need for your own belt. What a nice break! So you can slip into them as easily for a poolside margarita party (pairing them with an understated pale pink button-down or lace tank) as you'll slip into pajamas when you are ready for bed later that evening. For after a few ladylike runs into Tequilaville, you just *might* just find yourself sleeping in them, and comfortably.

BE TRUE TO YOURSELF (AND YOUR SIZE) The linen pant should fit comfortably on your natural waist or slightly lower, skim the hip and backside with a smidge of room, and have an airy float around the leg, offering a slight break at the foot. What's the reason the fit is so important on such a loose, easy pant? Linen has a tendency to lose its shape as you wear it and keep the impression of your seated shape—long after you have gotten up. So to avoid views of you with an oddly saggy bottom, hips that look magnified, and the elephant leg look, be sure that your pair fits you with perfection *before* you invest.

*Perfect
Partners*

page 55

page 26

page 171

page 166

page 217

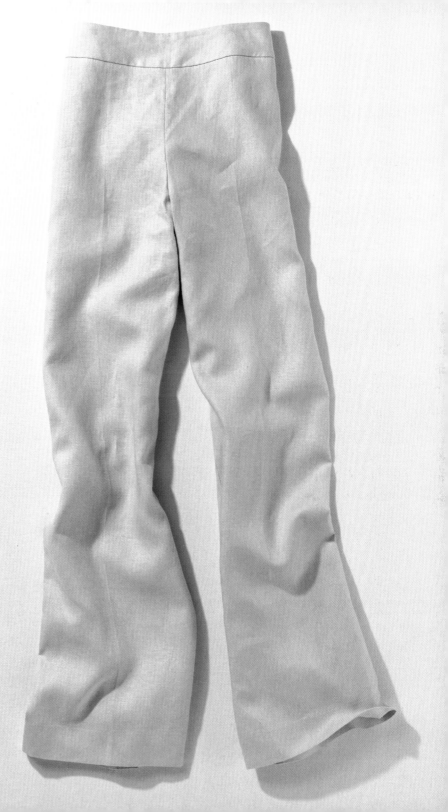

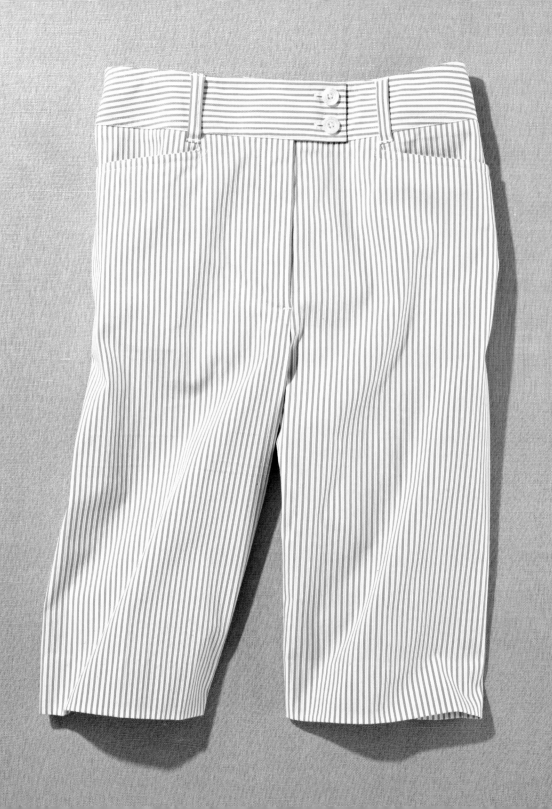

Ladies all over the world have embraced this traditional English walking short. They are usually slightly fitted to the leg and stop just a smidge above the knee. And whereas they were historically worn with knee socks and tailored jackets, today's Bermuda shorts remain classic, while boasting just enough modernity to make them believable for everything from work in casual warm-weather-based offices to weekends when you want to look active but not be in running shorts.

When you are ready to add the right pair, here is the

THE BERMUDA SHORT

long and short of what really matters most.

PETITES BEWARE Shorter women need always choose Bermuda shorts that skim the *top* of the knee, to maximize the visual length of your legs. If you want more coverage, choose a "cocktail length" *pant*, which goes down to just above the ankle. A short or pant that falls anywhere in between is in a visual danger zone.

JACKETS REWIRED A little suit goes a long way. Think about those casual weddings that pop up in the summer, that quick girlfriends' getaway, or those impromptu deck cocktails for a mix of friends and coworkers. This is exactly when you say hello to those around you in a smart Bermuda short and lightweight tailored jacket combination. Whatever your short color is, add a jacket in solid white and a matching white top, and you are fabulously finished, fast.

WORRY NOT "I hate my legs." "I don't look good in shorts." And if you think you look bad in *shorts*, there is actually nothing that looks worse than a woman hiding in plain sight, wearing long pants on the hottest day of the year—when the world around her is enjoying shorts. Pick your poison. It is time to just go ahead and enjoy the party, especially if you are hosting it!

Perfect Partners

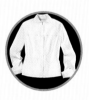

| page 34 | page 59 | page 78 | page 205 | page 161 |

Yes, pajamas. You can never be too prepared. Own a classic, stylish pair of "grown-up" pajamas for unexpected guests. I do.

Women's pajamas is a near $4 billion industry in the United States alone. I give some of the credit to Oprah Winfrey, who single-handedly put little-known pajama designer Karen Neuburger's "all day" pajamas on the map in the 1990s by exclaiming to the world that they were one of her "favorite things."

THE "GROWN-UP" PAJAMA

Here is a short list of nocturnal buzzwords that will kick your sleepwear choice into high gear.

FABRIC One hundred percent Egyptian cotton is the best to invest in, or cozy cotton poplin pajamas when you want the look and feel for less. Sea island cotton is a nice middle-ground fabric that will last and keep you feeling cool and cozy under warm bedding. Wrinkle-resistant cotton pajamas are also available today, but for what reason? Who knows?

BUTTONS Look for mother-of-pearl buttons. Cheaper, plastic buttons may crack over time from tumbling dry, leaving you with the chance of a sharply interrupted slumber.

COLOR White gets the vote for your first *good* pair of adult pajamas. Remember how you felt when you slipped into your last set of amazing white hotel sheets? That crisp finish, cool-to-the-touch hand, and soft sweep against your bare skin—you can get that without ever checking in when you choose quality white cotton sleepwear. And when unexpected morning guests pop up, you will look fresh and be ready to serve mimosas and scones like a timelessly chic host. No more apologizing for that worn-out college sorority T-shirt.

DETAILS A drawstring waist allows for total comfort and flexibility if your waist decides to shift sizes. And a fun chest patch pocket gives a sexy look, like you've borrowed your top from him. Many better cotton pajamas come with a matching storage bag in the same fabric, making your private ritual just a wink more special when packing for a trip.

Perfect Partners

page 26

page 171

page 59

page 217

page 214

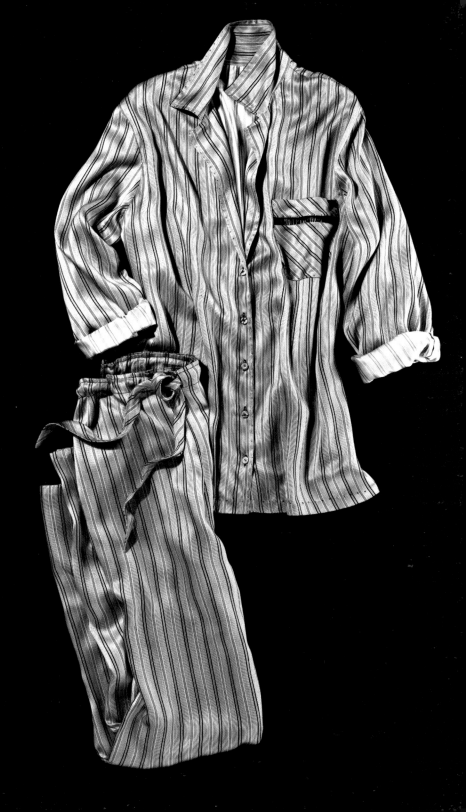

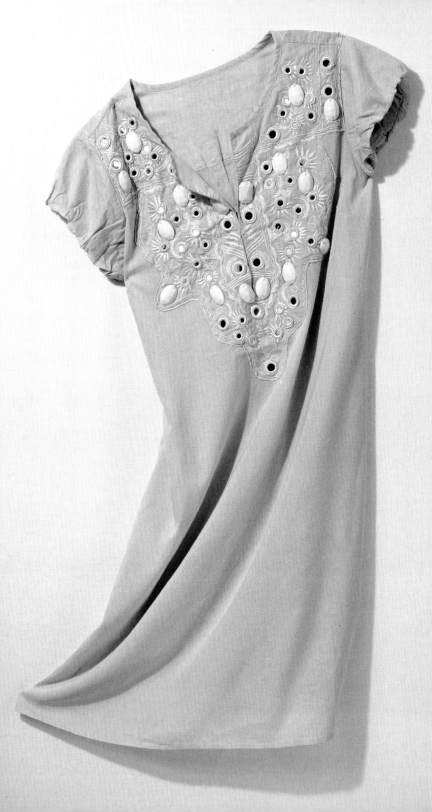

Perfect Partners

page 26

page 206

page 74

page 202

page 77

Depending on the city or town you live in, the dress you wear instantly puts you in a category. Let's take New York City, for instance. Women with sharply tailored shift dresses in black or charcoal gray and the stereotypical smart strand of pearls could very easily be pegged as Upper East Side. Whereas the sister sporting a long, tiered peasant dress, cropped denim jacket, and large hoop earrings might be a part of the new Harlem set. And let's not forget the classic New York chick who slips into her emerald green wrap dress, fashioned of a solid, clingy matte jersey—a clearly marked downtown girl who might be heading to work for a magazine, even.

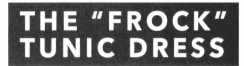

THE "FROCK" TUNIC DRESS

Every city has some kind of dress code, but the one dress that seems to baffle the system and flatter all ages is the "frock" tunic dress—a dress no woman should be without, especially for casual socializing.

THE TUNIC DRESS IS PERFECT WITH YOUR . . .

- best cropped tights layered beneath it and festive flats
- long-sleeve white T-shirt as a foundation and a wide belt to pull it all in

THE TUNIC DRESS IS CHIC AND UNEXPECTED WITH YOUR . . .

- fitted, cropped blazer, stacks of chunky jewelry, and ankle boots
- slimmest jeans underneath and a low-slung belt that hits you at the hip

THE FROCKY TUNIC DRESS IS QUESTIONABLE WITH YOUR . . .

- chunky heels and boxy blazers
- cowboy boots; some can, most can't

THE FROCKY TUNIC DRESS SHOULD BE AVOIDED WITH YOUR . . .

- sneakers
- hippie hats, moccasins, and the like

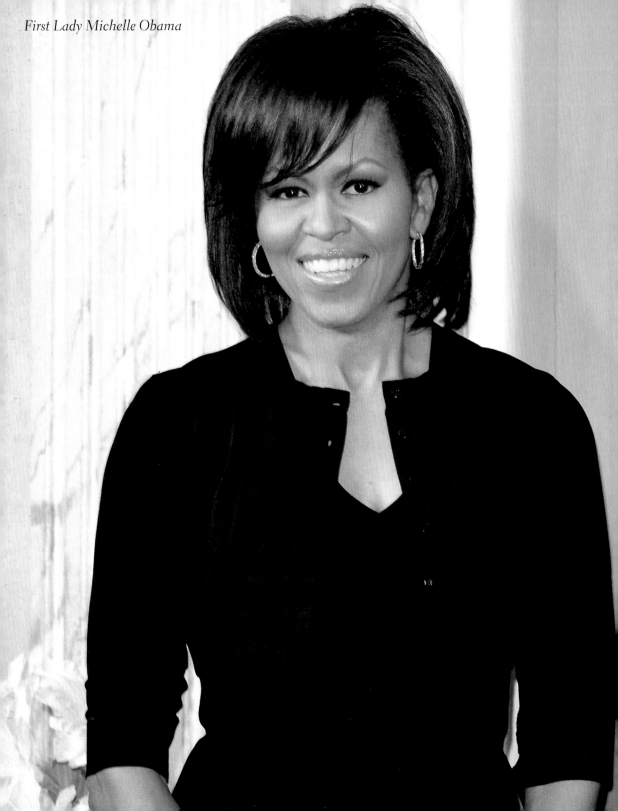

First Lady Michelle Obama

8 | POWER MOVES

M odern pearls, a talisman of sorts, mark the arrival of a lady. And no matter what room she enters, a woman adorned with a single or multiple strands of pearls shifts the attention of onlookers, inspiring them to sit up straight to receive her words, thoughts, and actions. Their effect is subtle but significant, mainly because of the iconic women most of the

MODERN PEARLS

world has seen wearing pearls before them and what they have represented in everything from politics to pop culture. Yes, they are an investment, but think of it as securing your place among a lineage of stylish women known the world over.

Princess Grace Kelly was known not only for her breathtaking leading-lady beauty, but for adorning her couture gowns with a simple, understated strand of pearls. This was in an era when women in high society tended toward more complicated estate jewelry. And there may not be a more iconic pearl-wearing movie character than Capote's Holly Golightly, as brought to the screen by the legendary Audrey Hepburn. Not to mention the powerful, *real-life* first ladies whose stately pearls took priority over fussy statement jewelry, such as Jackie, Barbara, and now Michelle. If anyone knows the importance of the power move in one's style vocabulary, it would be these women. Modern pearls seem to come along with the keys to the White House.

The most modern pearls aren't just a single strand of white cultured pearls. Today's pearls take on the personality of the woman featuring them. Here's how:

MODERN PEARLS	PERFECT WITH YOUR	CHIC/ UNEXPECTED WITH YOUR	AVOID WITH YOUR
Single-strand	fitted black pantsuit	black turtleneck	swimsuit
Double-strand	menswear shirt and pencil skirt	white T-shirt and jeans	ruffle-neck top
Stack of strands	red sheath dress	bohemian sundress and sandals	other necklaces

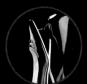

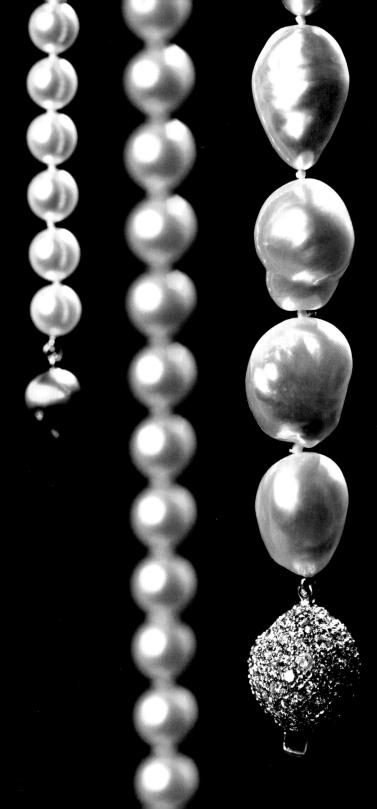

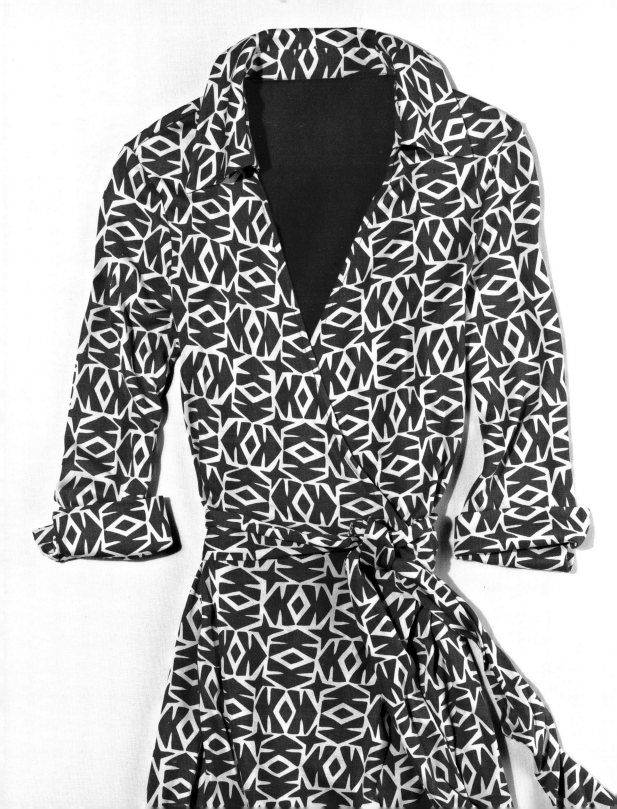

"So emblematic of 1970s fashion that it hangs in the Smithsonian Institution," said the *New York Times* of this figure-skinning garment. The iconic dress is the signature creation of Diane von Furstenberg. It remains available in her store as well as at upscale retailers around the globe.

The design is self-supported, not needing zippers or buttons. The look is polished but the feel is like a comfortable robe or a sexier kimono. Whether printed or solid, the wrap dress is a foundation of sorts, al-

THE WRAP DRESS

lowing the wearer to develop a look in a myriad of ways. The simplest approach to wearing the dress is to add sexy high heels, a slim minaudière bag, and earrings that dazzle.

Rock a more casual look with the quick addition of a medium-height espadrille or wedge, tote bag, and denim jacket or cropped blazer atop. But beware: Flat sandals make it look like a long workday has turned into a sad commute home.

"I've always been inspired by women, and my mission was to inspire women . . . the wrap dress made those women confident," says von Furstenberg. And although any woman can find one that works for her figure, she adds, "I would say the wrap dress is better when you are a bit curvier." Amen.

Let your first purchase be the three-quarter-sleeve version in black—especially if you don't already have a perfectly fitted, versatile black dress. Then get a bold print in color. You can layer a long, tissue-thin wrap sweater on top (secured with a wide or slim belt) or add a sharp white jacket with cropped sleeves—and opera-length leather gloves and knee boots (for cooler months). Experimenting with vamping it up is such good fun!

Perfect Partners

page 187

page 179

page 195

page 214

page 171

Jewelry can be a slippery style slope, adding hundreds, if not thousands, of dollars to your annual shopping budget if you let it. You can add bling in a stylish way without breaking the bank.

The best jewelry makes a subtle, more nuanced statement, allowing the *wearer* to remain the center of attention, not the accessory.

THE COCKTAIL RING

Consider the cocktail ring. It can add flair and an artful edge to your look.

As they say in the streets, "Go hard, or go home." This is the first rule of thumb, whether you are investing in precious metals and stones or costume options. Big, boldly cut, chunky cocktail rings make for elegant finishing touches that register clearly to the eye, take the place of multiple flimsy keepsake rings, and provide a giggle of color to more neutral clothing ensembles. So make it big and fun!

Warm amber, stately quartz, festive emerald, sexy ink, heavenly sapphire, sexy ruby, and the two "T"s, turquoise and topaz, top the list of stones that look amazing in überlarge cuts—even when you find a good-quality imposter. These classic tones never need match anything you are wearing and actually look *more* modern when they don't. These stone choices pair beautifully with silver, gold, or platinum settings, which allows for versatility and the ability to stand alone when you are not featuring other everyday jewelry.

If you are feeling *really* chic, take a cue from the past and pop your chunky cocktail ring on atop a sexy, fitted pair of black satin evening gloves. For real dazzle, work your ring with a bold cuff in the same metal as your ring (on the opposite wrist, of course) to allow for a yin-yang accessory moment when you need to revive anything from jeans and a tank to an easy sundress.

Perfect Partners

page 21

page 169

page 157

page 56

page 48

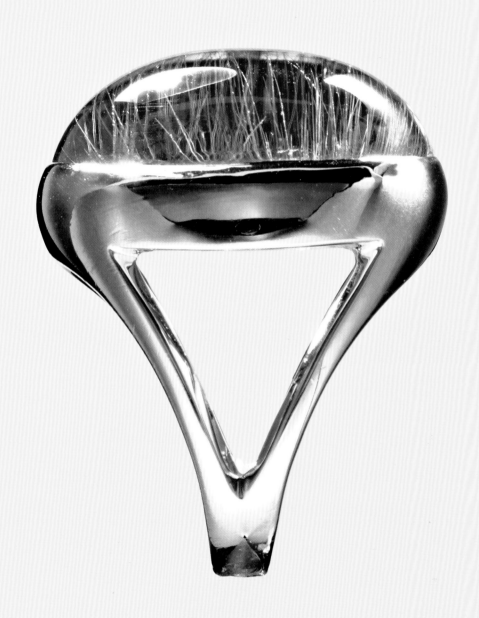

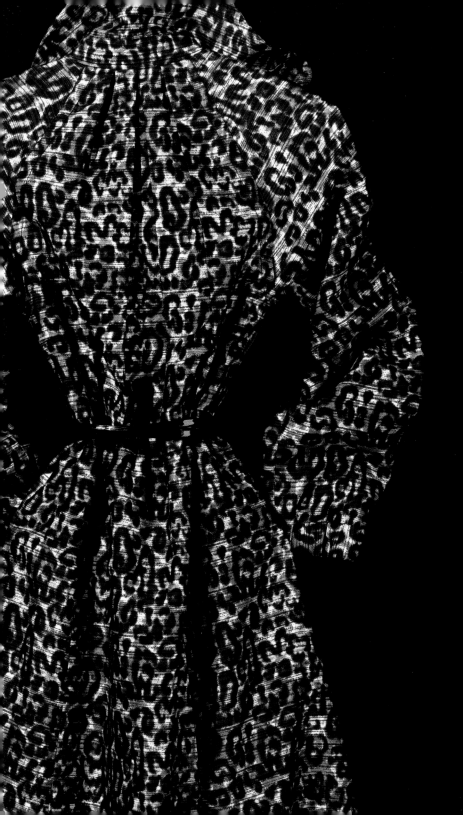

Women of a certain age remember the silver-screen starlets of the 1950s slinking into animal-print clothing without it being overly sexy—just cool. Sophia Loren's modestly cut faux tiger coat would get the paparazzi clicking just as fast as the next cleavage-baring actress. Today, the design duo Dolce & Gabbana is known for using animal prints as a *neutral* part of their collection, any year and almost any season—their customers know that it matches nothing, so it complements virtually everything!

THE ANIMAL PRINT

When you are ready to embrace this long-standing tradition of high style, select one single piece as a toe in the water toward "growl power." Make certain the item you reach for flatters you where you are in your life, as it can easily overpower a look if one is not careful. Here are easy ways to infuse the ferocious at any age.

TWENTYSOMETHING Animal cubs unite! The limit on wearing any print, from cheetah and leopard to zebra or giraffe, are far off in the distance. If you are a skinny girl try an animal legging beneath a solid tunic. Or push the envelope in a miniskirt in animal, which can boost a simple black jacket and black knee boots to new style heights. Take one bold piece and cool it down by making the others solids.

THIRTYSOMETHING A wrap dress calls out to you from the wild. Younger, slighter women might get swallowed up in such a full-bodied print. You, on the other hand, have seen a bit more of the world and are okay with the curves you've earned as a result. Since the statement will be a larger one (nearly head to toe), go red, black, or flesh-toned with your accessories to tastefully balance the look.

FORTYSOMETHING Run, don't walk, to get your hands on a fabulous animal-print trench coat or topcoat of great quality if you haven't already. This coat paired with a fresh white T-shirt and your best black pants gives the look of having had style for decades.

FIFTYSOMETHING AND BEYOND Animal prints are old news to you. So go for the small accents. A sexy pump or kitten heel in faux leopard, that wide belt atop your cream skirt suit in exotic zebra, or maybe simply a long, silky scarf in a metallic animal print of your choosing with your best chinos and a crisp white shirt. This is style déjà vu done right.

The menswear pant resurges every few fashion seasons as a "hot trend" to watch out for. The most stylish women never let theirs slip into light rotation and trust in the power of their amazing ability not only to artfully cover the leg, but also to provide a clever twist on the average female pant silhouette. Fuller, slightly wider, sometimes cuffed, and always with a pronounced drape, the menswear pant adds contrast and tension against the more feminine side of any woman's closet.

THE MENSWEAR PANT

The chic set will don it as a jaunty juxtaposition, feeling every bit of the danger and sexiness that come with bending the rules. Kind of like rolling up the waist of your pleated plaid private school uniform skirt just as dad drove away, or switching into your mom's high heels around the house behind the babysitter's back. Something about *slightly* forbidden style will always send a strong, sexy rush up your spine if done right.

Petite women can work this pant style with a word of caution: Make sure the wide leg isn't exaggeratedly wide, fostering a stumpy look in your lower half. Full-figured women should invest in a few extra pairs when they find the perfect version, especially those with "proud" hips, the ones that steal the first glances away from your eyes. The wide-leg menswear pant, when fitted properly, can offset that situation in an instant when you are careful of checks, plaids, and stripes that hug too closely.

And, tall gals, rejoice, for this trouser trick can add proportion to thin stems by increasing your overall volume—without adding real bulk. A fabric that moves will alleviate any chance of eyes mistaking fullness for flesh.

"The average man is more interested in a woman who is interested in him than he is in a woman with beautiful legs," was Marlene's strong take on everyone in the feminine world around her wearing skirts when she scandalously opted for his very own slacks; she never looked back, but trust that fashion always does and will.

Perfect Partners

page 172   page 48   page 29   page 171   page 104

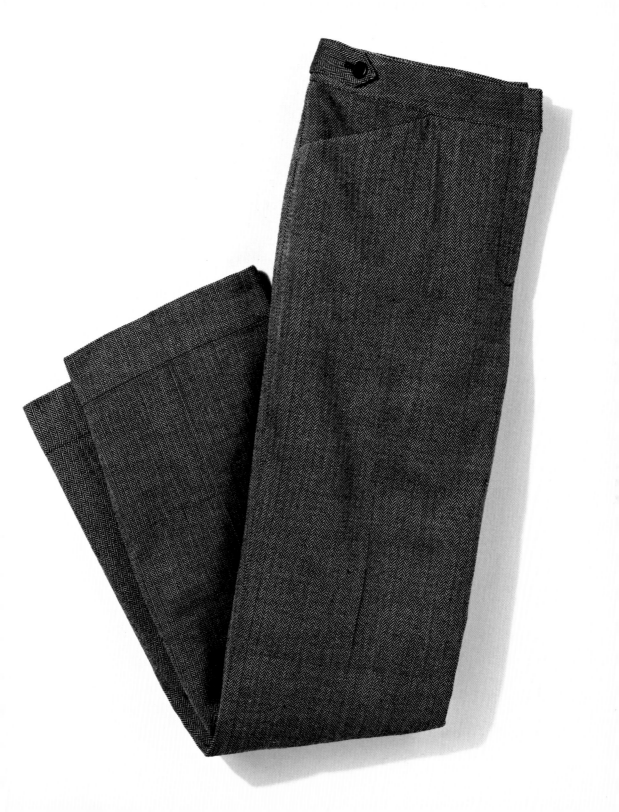

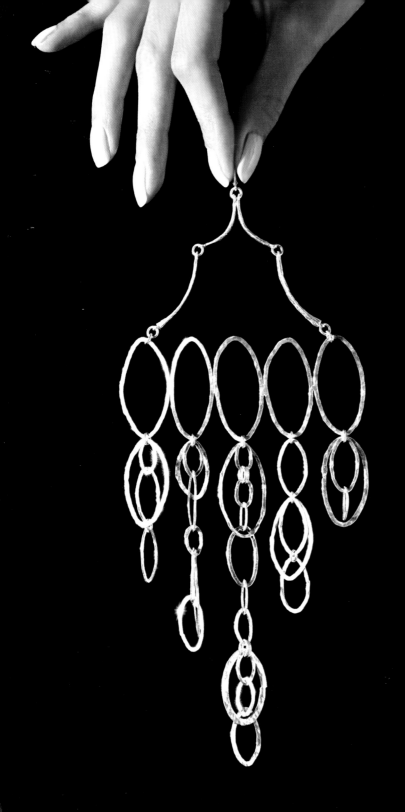

Perfect
Partners

page 3

page 192

page 180

page 217

page 161

The size and scale against the face, ear, and neck are what connote the epic status. Imagine what Elizabeth Taylor as Cleopatra may have worn. Or recall the earrings that stole each scene when you first watched *Sex and the City*, when chandeliers made their big return to fashion in the early part of the new millennium, after a seemingly thirty-year-long absence.

THE EPIC CHANDELIER EARRING

For not since their first modern heyday, with the 1920s' elongated art deco styles, followed by the 1960s' Cleopatra-inspired versions, had we seen the signature cascading design gain such global popularity.

The chandelier earring is not a safe choice. That's what makes it so fabulous. It signals that you are not another rank-and-file woman who chooses the appropriately scaled earring trend du jour. You can wear yours tonight, and on a special night ten years from now your ear candy will still be a classic.

Yes, chandeliers with gemstones are fabulous, but faux jewels work just as well.

The earrings should dangle, but not so much that they brush your shoulders. Even the slightest pooling of an earring on your body can look like a slovenly style misstep. For a nominal fee, a good jeweler can adjust or remove a bottom link if you fall in love with a pair that visually weighs you down.

If a pool party turns into a nighttime cocktail hour, pop them on with your swimsuit, your hippest cover-up, and sexed-up heels for a quick party-girl look (at any age). When business turns into pleasure and your work suit has to do double duty from conference room to cocktails, chandeliers can boost your basic tank and work pants when you ditch the jacket. Hair goes back or up (or off if you keep a spare), and the epic chandelier earring picks up the slack.

The trick to finding a truly epic pair is simple. Just when you think you have spotted a pair in a jewelry case that is big enough, push yourself to choose the next size up! If you stay in your comfort zone, you are guaranteed to look the same as you did the last time you got dressed up. Yawn.

Whether you choose vintage, new, or even a quality "inspired" version, your purchase of a Chanel jacket will honor the spirit of a female design legend who took many of her cues from the backs of men.

She liberated women from the corset in the early 1900s. Known for her infamous strength in both the design room *and* the boardroom, Coco Chanel offered not just a free-

THE CHANEL JACKET

ing take on daywear but a design point of view that remains internationally relevant and chic to this very day. She felt that "luxury must be comfortable, otherwise it is not luxury." The Chanel jacket might just be the tentpole of this very idea. From soft-cum-chunky menswear-inspired tweeds and jewelrylike buttons to nubby, supple bouclé adorned with sweet ribbons and dainty chains, the Chanel jacket as fashion icon is only surpassed by the little black dress.

Famous for its intricate construction and signature fit, the Chanel jacket is also a traveler's dream, as it dresses up or down without becoming wrinkled or shapeless. There are two great reasons to embrace this garment.

IT'S GOOD FOR BUSINESS This is the type of jacket to keep on the back of your office (or cubicle) chair. A black and white Chanel Jacket can be popped on over almost anything from a simple black shirt and white tank to a lavender shift dress, instantly pushing your ensemble toward "corner office," or to bigger and better no matter where you sit today.

IT'S GOOD FOR PLEASURE A Saturday trip to the car wash and farmer's market could turn into an early evening date night or pawned-off-theater-ticket moment with a simple text message or tweet. The Chanel jacket has your back. It's great with a low heel and a fresh white T-shirt. Your jeans, beat up or crisp, now have an elegant date too.

Perfect Partners

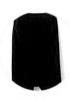

page 9   page 103   page 214   page 59   page 104

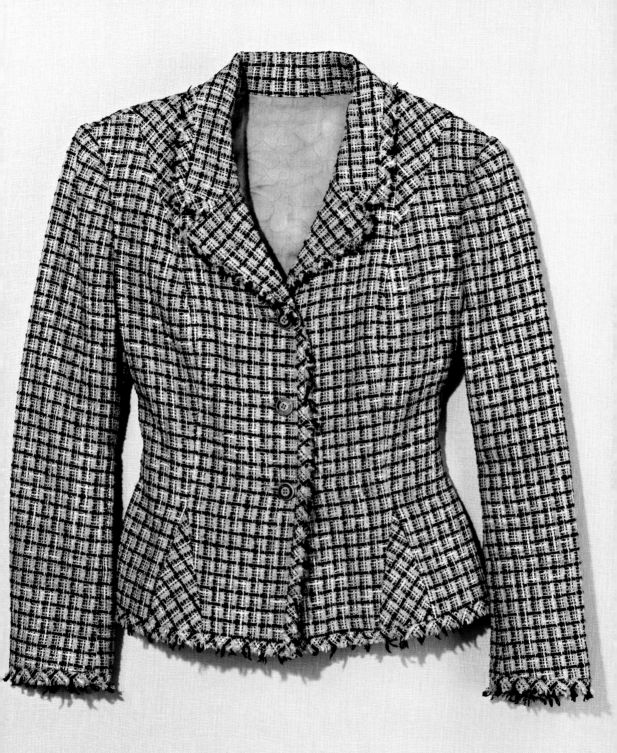

The color of fire, passion, desire, and strong energy, red evokes an alert intensity that cannot be easily duplicated with other warm colors. There is something that is unmistakably raw and regal about certain shades of red. The cheeky-cum-youthful glow of tomato red that almost vibrates to the eye, a wonderful glimpse of the red of a candy apple with its glossy finish inviting you to sweet surrender, or the globally recognizable fire-engine red—cooler to the eye with hidden hues of blue—can rev up a randy response in almost anyone, when used in the right setting.

THE POWER OF RED

Do we need to even mention a bold red lip color? This is Style 101 for most modern women, but if you skipped that class, here is a refresher. "The trick is choosing the right shade for *your* skin, and more importantly the technique—that's everything," according to celebrity makeup artist and beauty expert Cynde Watson. "Start with your bottom lip, directly from the tube—then mesh your lips together. Really press it into the lips so that it lasts longer. Take a lip gloss and add it to the top with a fine applicator to line the line perfectly—no liner pencil necessary. You can still wear color on the eye, just keep it subtle," she adds.

Harnessing that same power goes well beyond your maquillage; it makes its way seamlessly into clothes and accessories. When done right, a small dose goes a long way. It is the glints of red that make the most impact: the red soles of a pair of killer black heels that playfully attract the eye from across a room, the crimson lining of a handbag that flares to the eye when it's time to refresh your fragrance, or just the scarlet edge of a bra strap that peeks from beneath a strong power suit—but never all three. Use it like a secret weapon that adds danger to a seemingly safe vantage point. Here are timeless styling tricks to point you in the *red* direction.

WEAR	THE OKAY CHOICE	THE FABULOUS CHOICE
little black dress	black patent pumps	pepper red stilettos
white jeans and T-shirt	ballet slipper pink polish	candy apple red polish
navy blazer and tan pants	white blouse	red and white striped T-shirt
black pantsuit	skinny black belt	cherry red wide belt
dark-rinse jeans	black turtleneck	black turtleneck and red leather jacket
khaki Bermuda shorts	pastel T-shirt	oversize red linen shirt

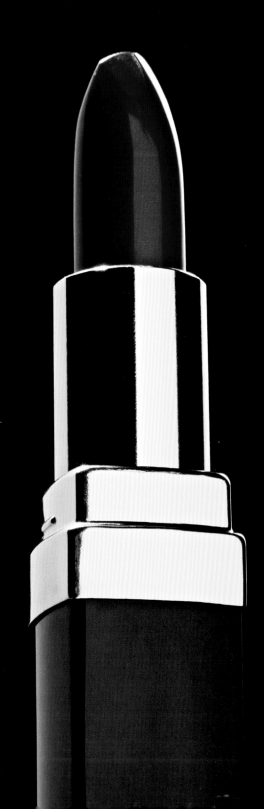

Perfect
Partners

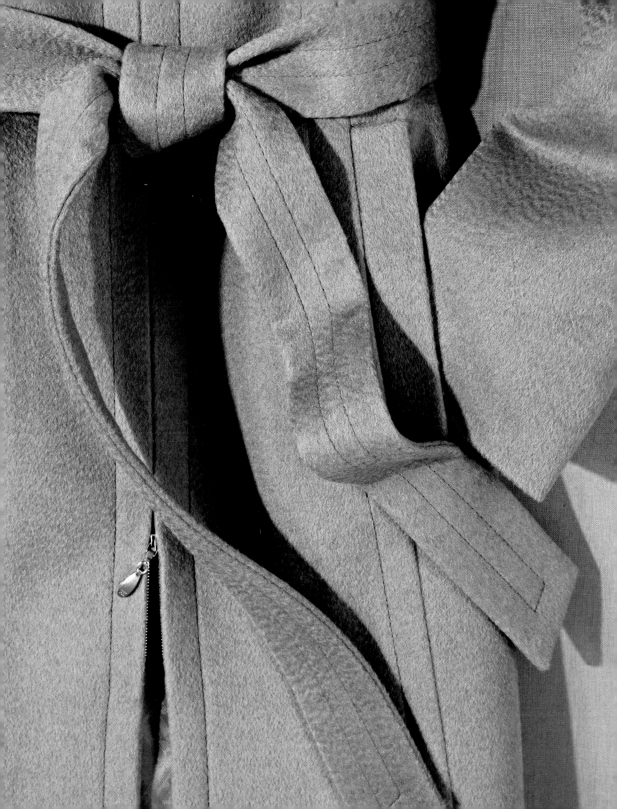

A coat that signals authority in an instant, signifies an air of comfortable confidence (not arrogance), and borrows a bit from the boys in its rich fabric, stately hue, and robust weight, the camel coat is easily a triple threat—if not a multiple style attack.

Historically speaking, the camel coat was known as such because of its camel hair fabric, which was, in fact, made mostly of hair from camels. This expensive process made for an even more expensive coat, leading many of today's designers and outerwear manufacturers to offer "camel" coats that draw

THE CAMEL COAT

on the original fabric and its signature color but are more modern versions created from fabrics that are blends of the animal's hair with fine wools. A staple season upon season from top designers and brands around the globe such as Ralph Lauren, Max Mara, Jones New York, and Brooks Brothers, this iconic idea has been translated from traditional buttoned models with strong peak lapels (think a foppishly worn coat à la that of Annie Hall) to renditions that wink toward modern with hidden zippers and modified funnel necks (offering a more feminine take, unifying perfectly with skirts).

The most special part of a good take on the camel coat is the sweep! That magical moment that happens as you walk in the open air, or even into a room with purpose. So take a cue from stylish women everywhere who make their camel coats become more personal. The Frenchwomen who belt their coats with thick, wide black belts. A *Grey Gardens* moment that few will try but the most stylish eyes will instantly laud. Italian dames who have worn them for decades with the collars pulled high, dark tights peeking out from beneath, and Sophia Loren–scale sunglasses that bolster the mystery. The stylish New York and Chicago power brokers who break out their camel coat just as the streets get nippy, adding a singularly poetic silk scarf, snug beret, and knee boots, riffing on a strong, spartan, military finish that amazingly still reads as sexy and feminine.

Perfect Partners

page 60   page 56   page 77   page 17   page 92

Vintage clothing and accessories are what separate women who turn heads from women who simply turn to the next hip trend.

A stylish woman's closet is truly a collection of varied expressions, emotions, feelings, experiences, and life tools translated into clothes and accessories. She takes a curatorial approach to editing the endless options that could suit her and artfully selects only the finds that

THE VINTAGE CONVERSATION PIECE

add visual value while preserving the continuity of her image. The vintage find would be part of a woman's "permanent collection," like the *Mona Lisa* at the Louvre Museum in Paris. It's not going anywhere. And it doesn't have to be just *one* find. The idea of a find is that it is special, haloing the more practical garments and accessories you might feature from day to day. This can be done with many different elements head to toe.

Some lean toward the quirky, taking the more obvious side of vintage goods to heart. Imagine a sequined bolero jacket from the late 1950s that the fictional Auntie Mame may have worn to float down her winding staircase, greeting guests at one of her legendary parties. Other, more modern women look for nuanced vintage, incorporating a touch of Yohji Yamamoto's signature "Pleats Please" pleated clothing collection from the early 1990s (which is now considered vintage to purists) into their current wardrobe. And if the aforementioned is still too much, imagine a gorgeous lipstick case from your grandmother's own collection passed down to you. Each time you pull out today's sheer lip color du jour during an elegant evening to reapply, the moment winks back to your lineage and the many places and swanky events where she may have done just the same with her signature jungle red.

The trick to nailing the vintage find is finding your signature vintage moment in time and sticking with it, more or less. Make sure it has a clear vision, like an area of a museum exhibition. Each decade past has several layers of style and design, and when you attempt to experiment with too many, vintage runs the risk of becoming comical.

When all is said and done, your look will be well worth the journey, for no one else is likely to have it, and everyone will want to know where you got it—thus its conversation-starting nature. As the curator of your own style, you will now be completely justified in simply saying, "This old thing?"

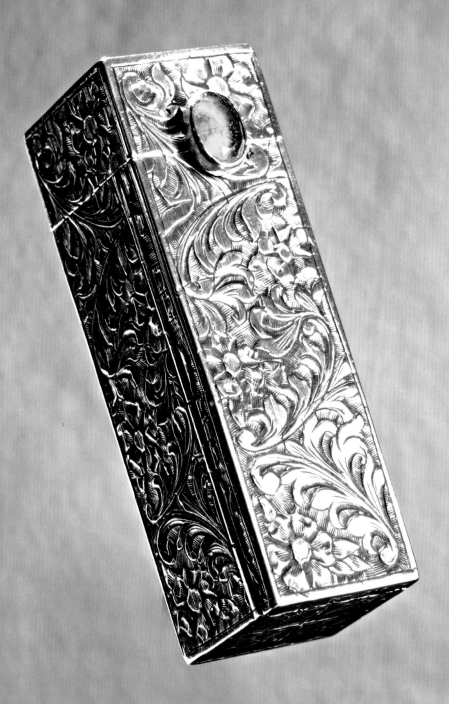

Perfect
Partners

page 69

page 56

page 107

page 59

page 95

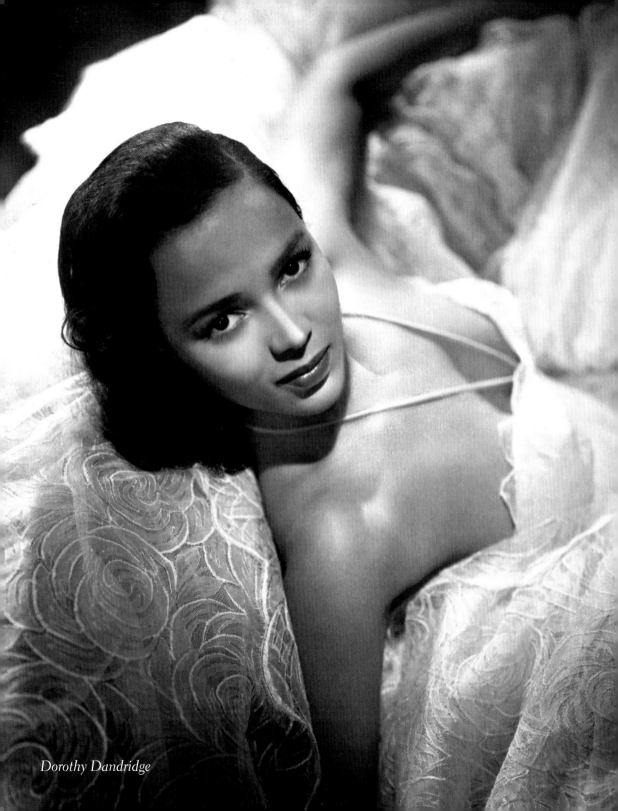

Dorothy Dandridge

9 | EVENING

R easons to embrace the metallic evening shoe:

THE METALLIC EVENING SHOE

BECAUSE THEY (AND WOMEN) HAVE COME A LONG WAY, BABY! Some women are still holding on to old-fashioned stigmas that associate certain shoe materials, like metallics, exotic skins, Lucite or acrylics, and even bold colors, with "ladies of the evening." Luckily, today's *modern* style seeker knows that this couldn't be farther from the truth when addressing chic metallic heels for evening, especially. First Lady Michelle Obama donned a pair in stark contrast to her emerald green dress at a White House event during *her* first one hundred days. And my friend the ever-so-stylish (and conservative) Elisabeth Hasselbeck can be seen proudly donning gold satin d'Orsay-style shoes with the big, sparkly baubles any given day of the week on *The View*. Two smart, strong women with very different platforms, both happy to stand in the same sparkly ones!

BECAUSE YOU'LL *FEEL* LIKE A STAR If you change nothing about your evening attire, adding a sexy metallic shoe will make even your most basic tailored black pantsuit look closer to a star's take on a tuxedo in a pinch. Pop the collar, swap your blouse for a flesh-toned or black camisole, add a smoky eye, and you are out the door looking fabulous! Why stay in life's background? It is time to pick a side: star or extra. You choose.

BECAUSE YOUR CLOSET IS SIMPLY BORING WITHOUT THEM There are moments when polite explanations just begin to sound like Charlie Brown's teacher spewing hornlike noises. If you don't own a pair of sexy metallic evening shoes by now, your closet is missing real punctuation that will get you nothing but compliments. Period.

Perfect Partners

page 184

page 188

page 166

page 217

page 161

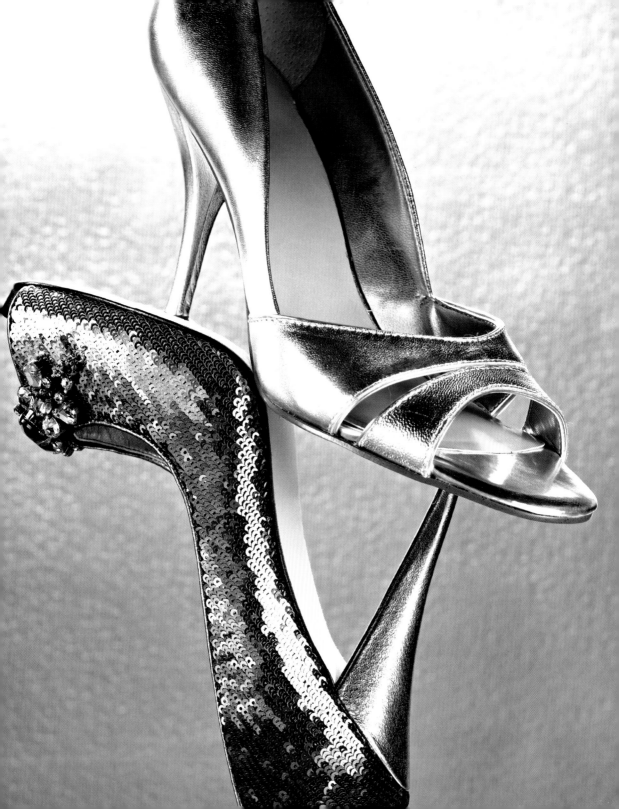

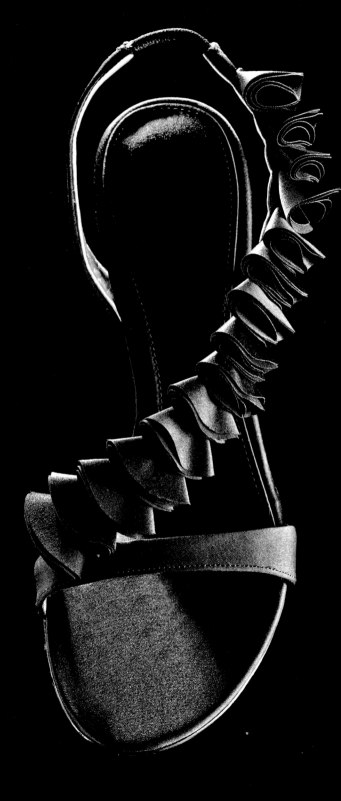

Perfect
Partners

page 195

page 21

page 9

page 171

page 202

Many elements of a masterful wardrobe can quickly transition from day to night, or desk to dinner, as some professional women may think of it. A classic black business pantsuit magically becomes a cousin to a tuxedo when paired with a shimmering wrap shell, drop earrings, and a long satin clutch. But your career pumps or flats usually have a tough time passing for nighttime shoes and instantly become a telltale sign of a look that screams, "She must have just run out of the office."

The most stylish evening shoes stand alone for a few reasons, the

THE EVENING SHOE

first being their stance, followed by decidedly artful design. High heels are traditionally the most appropriate choice, but thankfully, lower heels with a slimmer design, such as the half-inch kitten or Sabrina heel, are certainly equally acceptable and equally exciting to onlookers if they boast sassy-enough details.

The design details that speak to an evening affair have a leisurely elegance that partners with social nights filled with light feet, "no sweat" dancing, chatty mingling, easy circulating, or just posing in a chic collapse near the fireside. Imagine crystal embellishments, the tiniest of rhinestone beading, metallic straps that tie sweetly and dangle, bold satin bows, or cascading ruffles that give the foot a fashion gift-wrap for a special date to have fun unwrapping. And when paired with the perfect fresh pedicure, this is a true evening look, as luscious and decadent to the eye as a tempting dessert.

Unlike decades ago, when shoes were expected to perfectly mirror the color of your handbag or belt, the most stylish women today opt for burnished metallic finishes that align stylishly with anything from neutrals to bright clothes, bold strappy high-heeled sandals in black or a flesh tone welcoming the sweet or seductive dresses, or a vampy red or black ruffled shoe in satin or patent leather that brings heat to anything in noir, white, or neutral. Investing in a singularly perfect evening shoe might be one of the simplest wardrobe building blocks, as today it really shouldn't match anything you own. So scout for it on its own merit.

The true test of an evening shoe is its ability to make you stand a bit more confidently before you leave the house and part a crowded room with all eyes on you from the ground up.

Keep them stored sacredly, so they stay the way they were when they wooed you. Nestle them in a felt shoe bag for travel, secure them onto cedar shoe trees between wears to absorb moisture and retain shape, and be steadfast in restricting yourself to wearing them only for evening events when you barely need step on pavement, if you can. And they will never let you down and always lift you (and your outfit) up onto a pretty pedestal.

Add the cream dress pant to your style vocabulary. Not stark white and not too warm a cream, just the perfect shade of white with a just droplet of an amber glow diffused in. If found in a year-round fabric such as a tropical-weight wool, this single bottom has the unique power to allow you to create looks that speak to many classic style themes. Even if you don't see them celebrated in your favorite fashion magazine this month, have no fear.

THE CREAM DRESS PANT

Take note of my top five classic combinations that all star the cream dress pant, and know that you can fall back on them in any season with complete confidence—even when everyone is saying that the must-have neon green trench coat is back. Yikes!

CLASSIC THEME	PAIR THESE WITH YOUR PANTS	ACCENTED WITH
nautical	navy blazer and striped sailor T-shirt	gold accessories
safari	tan trench or jacket, and army green top	cognac shoes and bag
spectator	black and cream Swiss-dot blouse	black patent pumps
preppy	coral sweater set and grass green ribbon belt	straw bag and nude flats
Euro-chic	black turtleneck and beret	red slim belt and heels

Perfect Partners

page 7   page 64   page 180   page 162   page 205

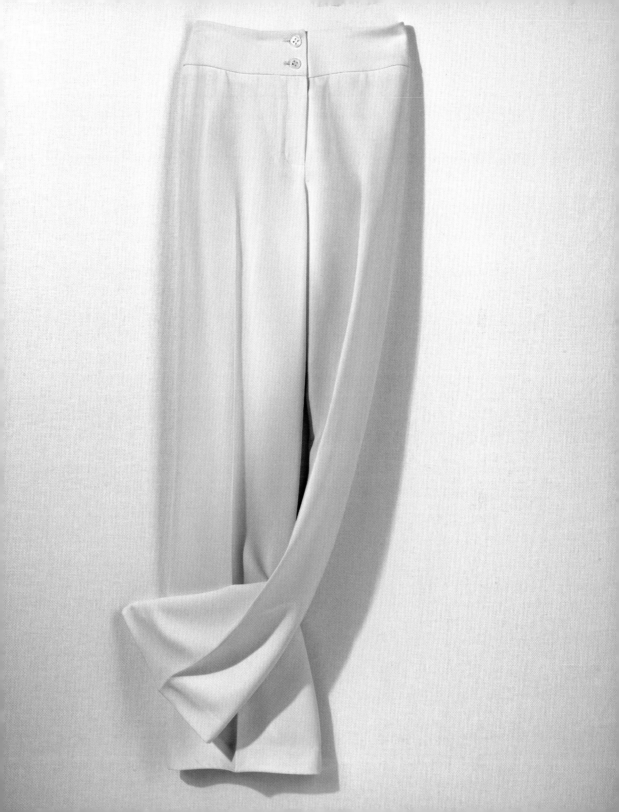

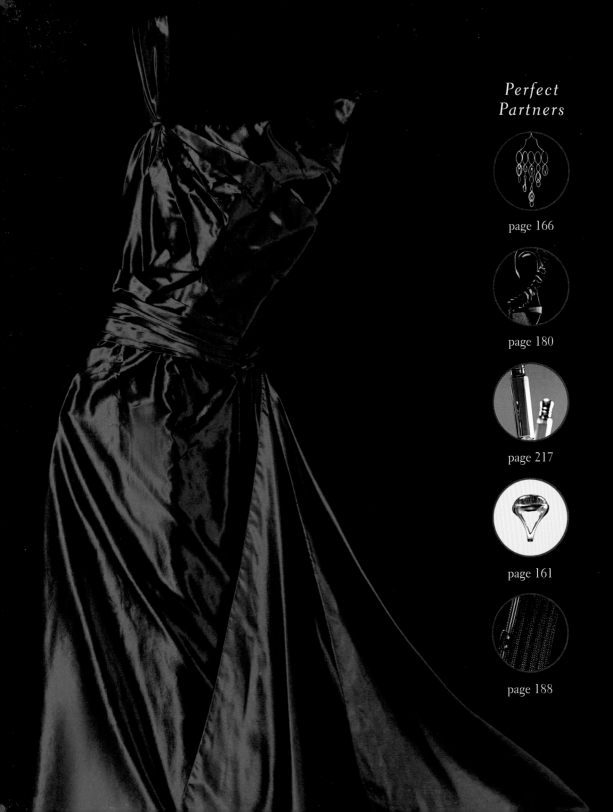

Contrary to popular belief, your little black dress *won't* take you everywhere. There are some occasions that simply require a more formal dress or gown, and the LBD won't be enough to just "get by." Even as casual as we have become in our modern-day society, a truly stylish and smart woman should have a tasteful evening gown in a somewhat traditional length on reserve.

Feel free to choose the dress that infuses a touch of a modern

THE EVENING GOWN

fashion statement and doesn't have the look of a dated cotillion debutante. Yet be sure to find it well before you need it. For there may be no greater shopping challenge (next to trying to find jeans or a swimsuit) than attempting to find the perfect evening gown under time constraints and duress. Can you say "*Ms. [insert your name here] regrets she's unable to make it*"?

Most women own a special *short* dress, either knee- or tea-length (about three to four inches above the ankle). This style expert finds that longer dresses are what are usually missing in most ladies' closets—unless they are the typical banished bridesmaid dresses that fill the *back* of many a cluttered closet.

Now is the time to rethink a dress in a longer length, one that revisits the brilliance and elegance of a time gone by. One in a sweeping cut that dances around the body and entrances those around you as you simply walk to refresh your drink. One that is ready *before* you are when it is time to get dressed for anything from a white-tie wedding or winter formal to a political or nonprofit fund-raising gala or red-carpet event even—hey, you never know. For the moment you say, "I will never be invited to a red-carpet event," is the exact moment you usually get the shocking invitation. Why not just be ready, having something on standby that isn't black, short, and off-the-rack looking.

The woman who lights up these types of events is usually the woman who flips the script and opts for an appropriate dress silhouette in a less-than-expected color with just a few subtle dips and surprises. Yes, select something versatile and somewhat nondescript that you can wear numerous times by just swapping out unique accessories, but don't choose black—go for a rich pewter gray, a deep dark cocoa, or even a classic ink navy. These tones are just as visually minimizing and appropriate as black but won't be as instantly identifiable as red, cream, or yellow (yikes!). As for a fail-safe fabric, silk taffeta is ideal, known for its timeless elegance and universal sophistication.

The black velvet blazer is the antidote for style panicking. For with items such as this, you will have no more crash shopping for big nights and simply learn how to make stylish shopping choices a part of your everyday life, so the pieces are at home just waiting for *you*.

THE BLACK VELVET BLAZER

Timeless, ageless, smart, chic, and sometimes sexy, the black velvet blazer gives a nod to equestrian-inspired riding gear while also being a staple of big-city women who desire a little luxe mixed in with their white-collar labor looks. An odd pairing of fan bases, but it works! You can see it everywhere from the collections of top designers like Michael Kors to more affordable brands such as Talbots.

Speaking of ageless, let's put this tried-and-true favorite to the test and see how to style it with fierce abandon at almost any age.

TWENTYSOMETHING Toss it atop that basic sheath dress, and secure it all with a wide belt in zebra stripes, even—regardless of the dress color. Add black opaque tights and black patent leather heels, and your evening starts the moment you turn your back to that stifling cubicle. And you will *own* all the party photos you've been tagged in on Facebook, thanks to the jacket's subtle shine, which attracts a camera flash.

THIRTYSOMETHING Classics, marry it to a fitted black trouser. Modernists, try pairing it with lean, sharp satin pants in charcoal gray. Trendy chicks, scrunch the sleeves, pop the collar up, and layer it with fitted jeans and a men's ribbed white tank top. As for the romantic, haul out a ruffled top, a skinny belt to go atop both, and finish it off with black knee boots and a full, flowing lace skirt.

FORTYSOMETHING Keep it *young* and avoid the look of a schoolmarm by wearing it with your more sporty bottoms rather than the dressy ones. Think denim skirts, fitted cords, cropped khakis, and even cargo pants!

FIFTYSOMETHING AND BEYOND Velvet has a rich look to it, and if it makes sense on anyone, it would be the women in your age bracket, who have earned the right to look and *feel* wealthy. This may just be with your clothes, but no one needs to know what's in your bank account. Make this era feel beyond luxe by keeping the blazer styled with a comfy-chic edge. My top three bottom prescriptions: a great-quality black yoga pant for travel, crisp white jeans for weekends, or fun plaid pants for the holiday season.

*Perfect
Partners*

page 192

page 21

page 214

page 180

page 171

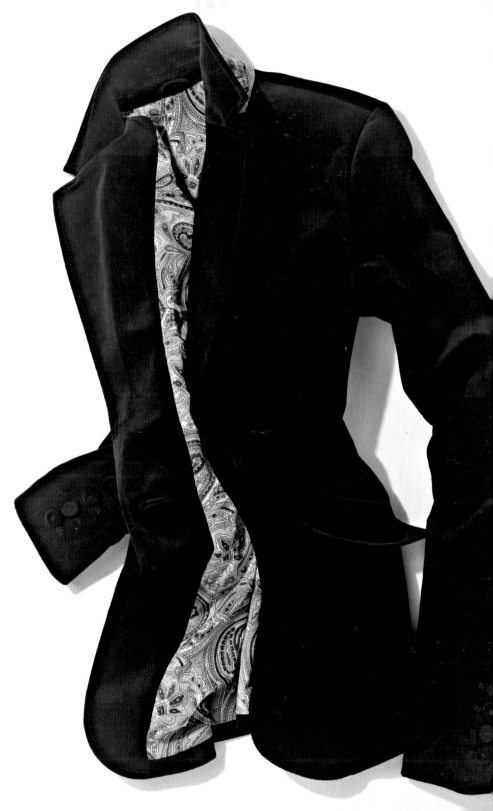

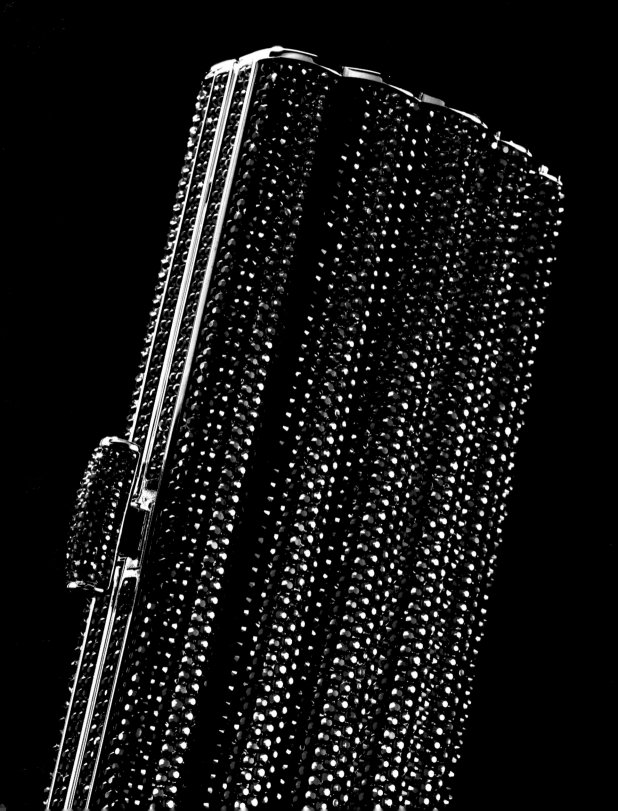

This bag should fit securely in your grasp, be it a long, slim minaudière trimmed in satin or a short, square envelope design that is finished in bugle beads. Picture an oversize clamshell in coral, a jewel-encrusted minaudière, or a lacquered bamboo stunner—let your imagination take over your desire to have function. For tonight, there should be little utility, just fabulosity and fun!

Art, craftsmanship, and finished details are what make others take notice—or not, for that matter, as some of the most beautiful

THE STATEMENT EVENING BAG

statement evening bags do nothing more than add an elegant whisper or a giggle to a more serious outfit, or subtly complete a perfect black dress and bold red lip combination. Yet it is still a statement, the right statement.

No need to have dozens of statement clutches if you are not in the position to invest in them or don't have any interest in sourcing them. Whereas most women see having only one of something as being doomed to "repeat offending," many trend*setters* and style aficionados view this "only child" approach to accessories as a way to develop a truly personal style signature. And there is no better statement than having your own signature style; this, you *cannot* buy.

Perfect Partners

page 136   page 9   page 17   page 214   page 217

The evening wrap can completely kill a look if it isn't chosen properly or wrapped elegantly. The one thing that women should realize is that the *modern* evening wrap is the one that brings an outfit to a sophisticated crescendo and does not create a cacophonous ending to an otherwise beautiful dress or ensemble.

THE *MODERN* EVENING WRAP

Women are the first to get cold in a room of dressed-up minglers, and you certainly have good reason. As we men sit in layers of wool jackets and cotton shirts, you shiver beside us in a sheer top, lace skirt, and open-toed sandals, having to look unfazed. Enter the modern evening wrap.

It is deemed *modern* for the simple reason that it is not your mother's, or worse yet, grandmother's, evening wrap. You know the one. Might feel like a thin lace piano shawl of the 1890s or a wimpy, tassel-edged pashmina reminiscent of the 1990s. Both of these add little or nothing to today's best evening looks. What I find that they can add—if you are not careful—is visual weightiness, an old-fashioned finish, and worse yet, years!

The trick is embracing the unexpected and being okay with something not technically being a wrap. Selecting something so unique that it stands on its own as art—so it never really matches anything exactly—simply complements your look of the night, or pops against it. It could even have sleeves built in, making it a shrug or sheer jacket of sorts that does double duty as a light topper *and* wrap. Look for the unforeseen solution that sets you *apart* in the room. This you may not find in your local department store along with your other basics; it may be off the beaten path in a small boutique.

If your town is in close proximity to a traditional East Indian sari shop, you have a gold mine of beautiful imported fabrics in silks or soft, sheer cottons, many offered in punchy colors with metallic threads that add shimmer and a festive tone. The subtle stiffness of the fabric holds its own shape and gives you the freedom to wrap it almost any way—without looking like you made a mistake.

Also investigate your local Chinatown, Koreatown, or even African fabric stores. You will find similarly exotic fashion fare that will elevate your wardrobe by adding a finishing touch that fuels conversation to your face, versus the old-school versions that may only inspire murmuring behind your back. That's just so high school.

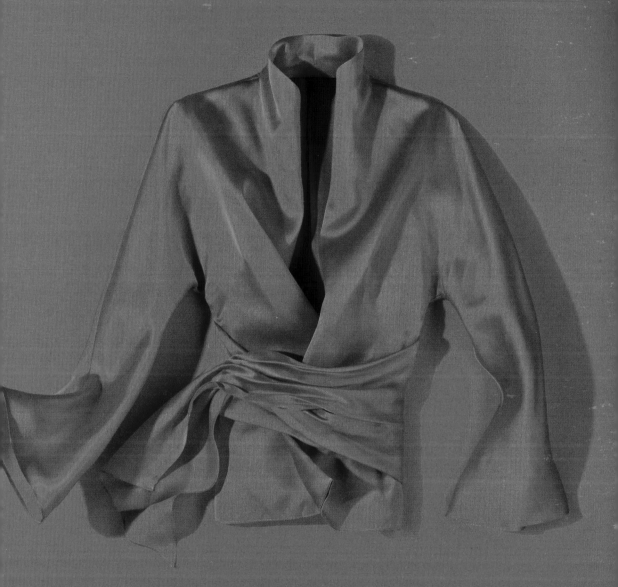

Perfect Partners

page 63   page 179   page 166   page 161   page 202

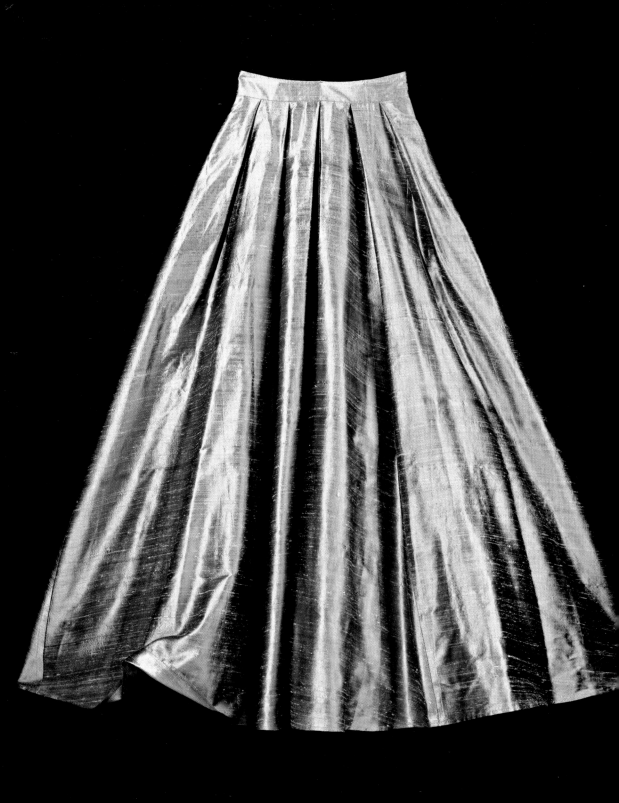

race Kelly and Dorothy Dandridge immediately come to mind when I see a lovely, fluid ball gown skirt that speaks of the 1950s, an era when starlets such as these put in the time to create the look and mood that we now know to be the proverbial red carpet moment—usually *without* the help of what we call today a "celebrity stylist." And there is nothing wrong with the practice of keeping a stylist in your back pocket, but when you actually *know* the essential items to keep on hand, especially for evening, who needs a second opinion or a runner?

This skirt is definitely one for your top ten list of

THE BALL GOWN SKIRT

evening style essentials; which other elegant classics have stood the test of time quite as well?

On the practical side, it can cloak the hips—without looking like you are trying. And its scale can make your top half appear slightly smaller.

Your first try at this skirt of legend should be a dark color that is versatile enough to be featured for several appearances without the risk of looking like you are repeating your one evening skirt again and again. I vote for a rich inky black, deep navy blue, or chocolate brown (in that purchase order). A beautiful duchesse satin or silk dupioni makes it regal, and a design with as few details as possible (avoiding any ribbons, ornamentation, etc.) allows it to be a silky blank canvas that welcomes a myriad of tops. Take a look at these top three ways to artfully complete a look stemming from any of the options above.

OCCASION	PAIR THESE WITH YOUR SKIRT	ACCENTED WITH
formal wedding	black skirt and pastel angora twinset	stack of pearls
outdoor gala	navy skirt and crisp white shirt (untucked)	a slim or wide belt
theater opening	brown skirt, pink blazer, and pink camisole	metallic cuff and heels

Perfect Partners

page 52

page 48

page 107

page 214

page 96

For the most potent style statement, select one that *contrasts* your wardrobe. For instance, if your closet is filled with neutrals, a juicy persimmon shawl-collared coat with dolman sleeves is just the right prescription. You may own nothing but solids, so a ladylike coat in an

THE LADYLIKE EVENING COAT

exploded black and white houndstooth, a colorful magnified tartan, or a racy animal print will rev up your predictable look while fighting the chill. Coats such as this will help casual chinos paired with a tank look dressier and look commensurate with your best little cocktail dress—unlike trying to pass off your straight, worn-out office overcoat as an evening coat. It never works.

And unlike your first girly coat, which most women don't remember having a say in selecting, your power to choose today's version is what will set you apart. Make the first one you run to the one you *don't* buy. Think outside of your usual wardrobe's palette boundaries, reverse your own norm, and imagine the girl you once *were*, the girl who took chances, wasn't afraid to play in her new clothes, and came home a little disheveled—yet still cute because of her fabulous coat. For it was that very free spirit that inspired bolder, fresh choices. Listen in, and honor your inner style child, if only for this one purchase, and you will always feel like a lady when you wrap up and head out into the cold.

Perfect Partners

page 183   page 21   page 64   page 202   page 214

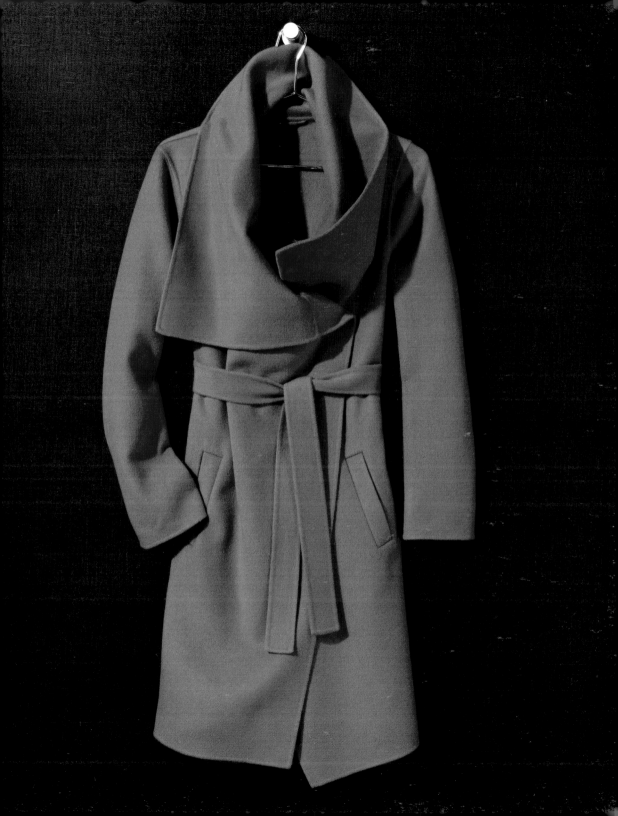

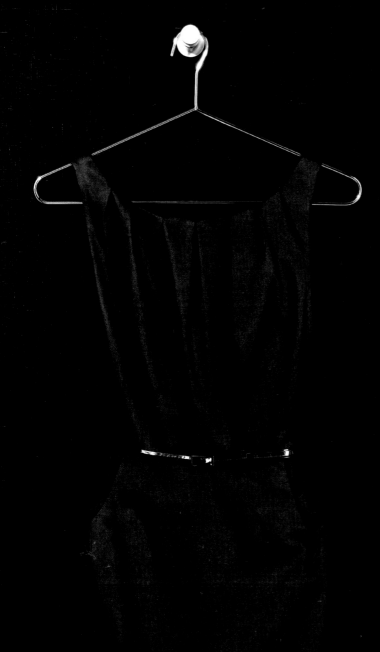

Perfect
Partners

page 144

page 171

page 166

page 217

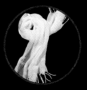

page 77

We know it, we love it. Take a look at four of my favorite ways to style the iconic little black dress at every age.

TWENTYSOMETHING Hopefully your version reveals as much of your arms and legs as you feel is appropriate—they won't ever look exactly the same in the decades ahead. A slightly above-the-knee sheath with generous neck and arm

THE LITTLE BLACK DRESS

openings will serve you well. Layer a thin white button-down beneath it for work, pair it with black textured tights and peep-toe pumps in a cool metallic tone, and finish off with black fingerless gloves and a white patent clutch. Pure heat!

THIRTYSOMETHING The dress you invest in should reflect your life trajectory ahead (not behind you), and whether personal or professional, the quality should be one and the same—great. Spend as much as you can stand, and just when you're at your limit, be prepared to add a bit more in tailoring. Wear it like a purist, and allow it to stand alone against sexy hair, glowing skin, and gams by Pilates! Breathtaking nude shoes, diamond studs, and one single bold cuff bracelet are all the accessories you'll need to pull it off like a minimalist.

FORTYSOMETHING This might be your third or fourth LBD, and the world should know that you have always understood its power when you slip into it. Now is your season for fun *and* fabulous styling. A belt will take you there (just ask First Lady Michelle Obama). For you, a wide or skinny belt in an exotic faux skin like muddled python, abstract cheetah, or iridescent ostrich can set the stage. Knee boots in black drive the sexiness home, and a cropped jacket or cardigan keeps this funky style equation sweet.

FIFTYSOMETHING AND BEYOND You might have a few more anxiety areas to conceal, so consider finding your dress of choice in the *knit* fabric family—not woven. Matte wool jersey is the first one to look for. Might it be a wrap-dress style? Yes, if you are top "heavenly" and bottom "blessed." Or maybe just a loose frock style that you can belt in good months and leave loose around the holidays. Any road you choose, add fun heels in anything but black, one strong statement necklace (think chunky ethnic, Lucite, or even multistrand carvings), and polish off the look with flirty, flesh-toned fishnets!

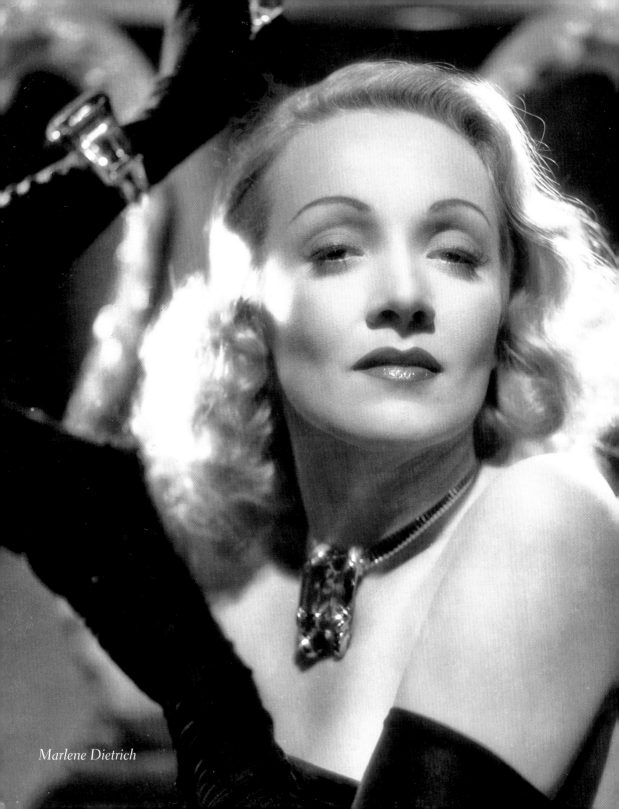

Marlene Dietrich

10 THE FINISHING TOUCHES

t is high time for women to come out of the style closet and at last be prepared to reveal their wallet with *total* confidence. No more fumbling for that debit card in the dark of your tote, for fear of the judgment set to befall you at the cash wrap if that tattered wallet sees the light of day. Gone are the days of quickly snatching your wallet from inside your desk drawer and tucking it under your armpit as you dash off to lunch with your officemates. If either scenario is you, your more sophisticated wallet is calling.

THE SOPHISTICATED WALLET

What you pull your money *out* of will dictate what kind of money you will ultimately put back *into* it. Those who look like they *don't* need wealth are usually the ones who garner it faster. Think about the gorgeous celebrities who rack up gifts and perks just because people are happy to have met them. Or consider the well-dressed job applicant who aces an interview in a perfectly appointed suit, with a dazzling smile, noteworthy handbag, and firm handshake—versus the disheveled candidate who has that slightly unkempt edge, digging for a dog-eared résumé while her cell rings aloud for the interviewer to hear. Your wallet, or "personal financial vessel," if you will, transmits a message to those around you about the time and care you put into your own matters of organization, money, and style. So, whether interviewing, entertaining a client, or about to split the check with a first date who might be "the one," be completely secure the next time you do the reach and pull for your wallet.

The most sophisticated choice to start your collection with is usually top-quality leather in a solid color. Remember, leather that is top-quality usually doesn't have a gold-embossed stamp that says so. And even if you never branch out into the more zippy snakeskin, jaunty bold-colored leather, or supple printed satin, you will always have a classic go-to wallet

Perfect Partners

| page 4 | page 113 | page 41 | page 85 | page 10 |

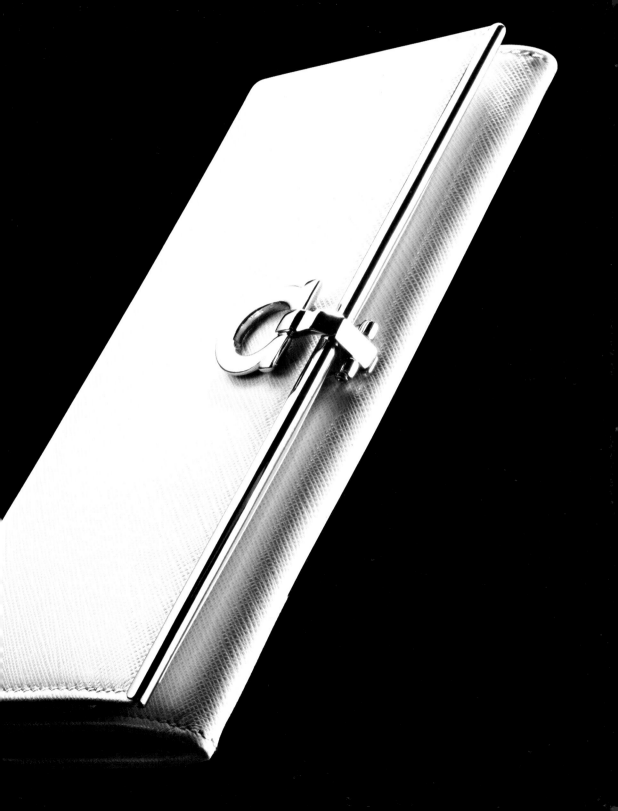

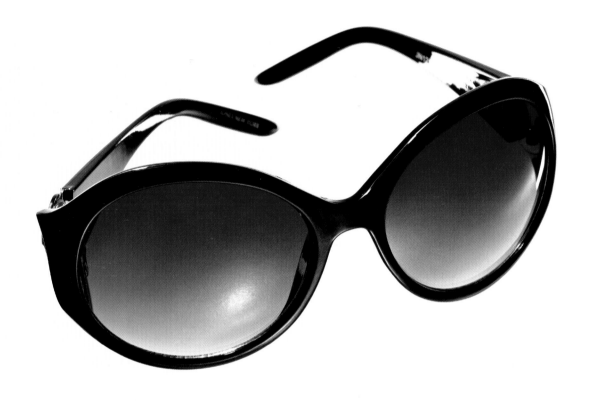

Perfect Partners

page 70

page 42

page 59

page 140

page 157

Every few years a notable woman will become even *more* of a style luminary because of her choice of sunglasses. Style watchers witnessed this in the 1950s as Grace Kelly, sporting her cat-eye lenses, ignited the paparazzi's flashbulbs from Hollywood movie sets all the way to her legendarily reclusive royal life in Monaco. The oversize dark Chanel frames donned by Jacqueline Kennedy Onassis became the trademark of a generation of women who emulated the same look in the

THE ENVY-INSPIRING SUNGLASSES

1960s and do so even today. And who could forget Madonna's Ray-Ban Wayfarer redux that defined the East Village pop-gone-soft-punk style of the MTV eighties.

Whether selected to hide a day sans makeup or be the dramatic curtain that reveals your most sparkling eye shadow and perfectly threaded brows, envy-inspiring sunglasses increase mystery while punctuating an artfully turned-out look.

In recent years, sunglasses have become de rigueur, nearly replacing the need for elaborate clothing and jewelry. The woman who leans toward minimal dress, featuring a basic solid button-down shirt in a pale color perfectly paired with a black pant and matching flat, can instantly complete her look with a pair of tortoise sunglasses and a bold lip color. No need for a belt, scarf, hair clip, anklet, or statement bag—especially if the sunglasses are beautifully crafted.

The most stylish women will have a few pairs on reserve to match their every mood. Larger and darker may be reserved for driving to events that require a strong, dramatic arrival. Smaller, rectangular frames with slightly tinted lenses in classic rose may be on standby for lunches or launches with ladies who take particular note of stylish details.

Invest in a quality single pair first. Push yourself to avoid bargain sunglasses you might be able to buy along with your toothpaste, hand lotion, and vitamin C tablets at the local drugstore. And the "steals" that you might be able to buy from a street vendor are probably just that: stolen. Take an hour or two, bring along an honest gal pal, and visit a retailer that offers labels you might not be able to pronounce—if only for fun. Take note of the sunglasses that make you feel like dressing up a bit more to complement them. Chances are, they will look great with jeans and T-shirts also. If you dare, invest at that moment, or go down in price, purchasing a similar version at a slightly less expensive retailer.

According to many historians, the classic circular earring design dates back to about 200 BC, originating in the Middle East and Asia, with pierced versions being credited to Egypt closer to 1500 BC. And whether used as a sign of wealth and prosperity or tribal initiation, the hoop was a centerpiece of adornment for men and women. They were unique artifice with a very distant correlation to the fashion accessories most know them to be today.

THE HOOP EARRING

Whether quarter-sized, teacup-brim-sized, or the classic version that measures just under an inch in diameter, hoops today can be found in, or custom-made in, the exact shape, finish, width, and material you desire. Smaller, mesh versions in sterling silver speak to the more traditional set, whereas gold renditions with the circumference of a tennis ball have attracted younger women with a more urban style sensibility (can you say JLo?). You can be an angel or a vixen in hoops; it's just in how you choose them.

The challenge with prescribing such an omnipresent element of the world's jewelryscape is making sure women know exactly when to opt to hoop and when to consciously decline. Take a gander at this style expert's hoop dreams for women everywhere and almost any occasion that may arise.

HOOP SIZE	PERFECT WITH YOUR	CHIC/ UNEXPECTED WITH YOUR	AVOID WITH YOUR
Scarsdale small	fitted pantsuit	black turtleneck	gym attire
Midtown medium	sexy jeans and white T-shirt	tuxedo pantsuit and camisole	infrequent dive bar nights
Bronx large	bohemian frock and sandals	poolside swimwear	little black dress

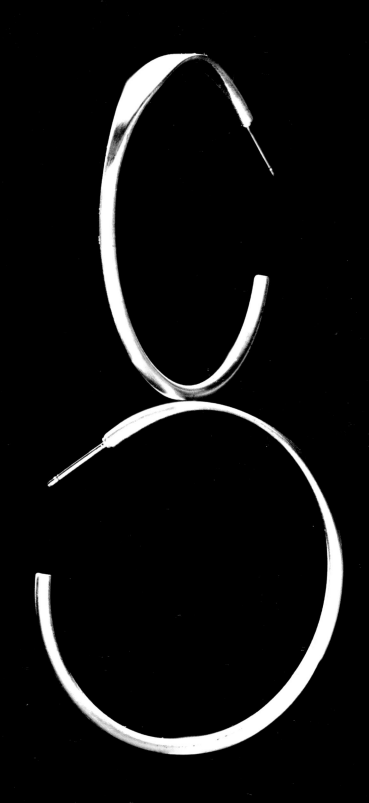

*Perfect
Partners*

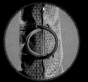

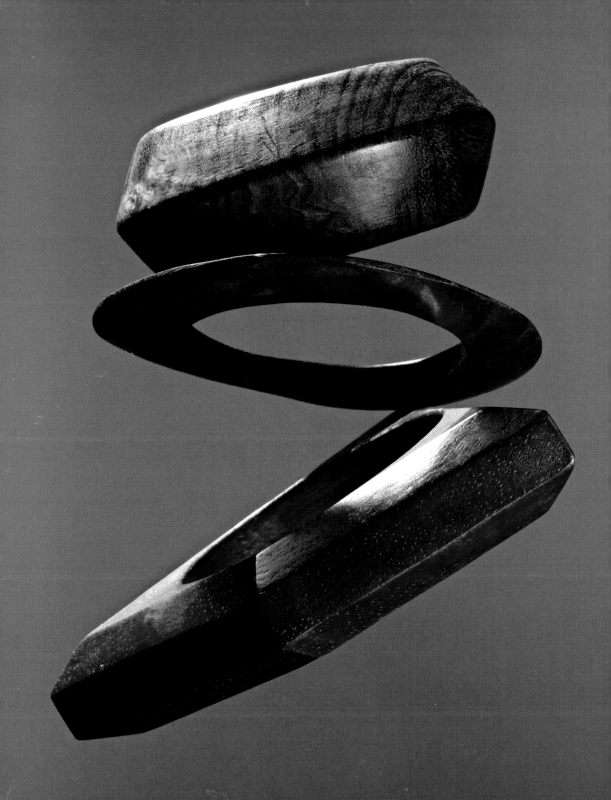

They are usually bold in design (spherical, thickly carved, tall in height), textural (stained, natural wood grain markings), and worn expectedly *and* unexpectedly—with anything from a classic tan safari jacket to a slinky metallic evening gown.

What makes the trio of wooden bangles a pure investment of lasting style is the fact that this wristed trifecta has been around since long before you—on the arms of many cultures, including Africans in Tanzania, who wear them in rich varnished black wood—yet will still be available today and tomorrow. And they will

THE TRIO OF WOODEN BANGLES

still be chic, whether on the mother continent or on the mother of all runways—New York Fashion Week—long after you are gone. Take this as reassuring though, for knowing what will live on in matters of style will not only arm you with more nimble shopping skills but give you accent assets such as these, ready to help you sparkle in an instant.

If the trio part scares you, as with your cocktail of choice, you can always opt for a single or make it a double. The more you add, the greater the impact on your overall look. Here's how:

WOODEN BANGLES	YOUR CLOSET CLASSICS	THE RESULT
black wood	crisp white shirt and black pants	No-brainer chic
pale wood	light blue shirtdress and flesh sandals	*Into* Africa
cognac wood	denim jacket and printed sundress	California soul
mahogany wood	medium gray pantsuit and wine shoe	Softer side of CEO
dark chocolate wood	dress in tangerine and bronze heels	Hermès on a dime

Perfect Partners

page 13   page 21   page 48   page 104   page 161

The umbrella you choose to hold is an immediate indicator of so much *more* than how dry you will be. Like the aforementioned details, it counts as a part of your accessory silo, and albeit in less-frequent rotation, it has a firm place for when you *do* need it.

Identifying what makes a good-quality *and* stylish umbrella is two different challenges. Top-quality designs can be found today in almost any department store nationwide, but are they

THE PERFECT UMBRELLA

stylish in terms of being a nonconformist accent, like a unique brooch or cocktail ring, occasional evening glove, or other infrequent bit of haberdashery? Whereas many of the more fashion-forward umbrellas that you see in bright candy-colored finishes or plaid prints of the moment may not necessarily be of the quality that weathers the storm. The best overall style would have to be the classic clear-canopy umbrella, a timeless marvel. For getting inspired to dress for the rain on a gray day is hard enough on its own. But why ruin a hard-to-create outfit that already is braving the elements with an umbrella that just blends in or covers it up? This style expert would rather prescribe for you an artful, discreetly patched up, vintage stunner with unique character any day, rain or shine.

Going vintage is one solution. Not only will you find an inclement weather fix, you will find the character, details, old-world weightiness, and individuality that click-and-gos from big brand names may not offer.

So whether you choose a fixer-upper or invest in a new model, remember that your choice will always be factored into your overall rainy day look. Making it count is also about making sure you understand that you're not just covering your head, but covering another carefully selected accessory addition for your closet.

Perfect Partners

page 82   page 9   page 187   page 103   page 59

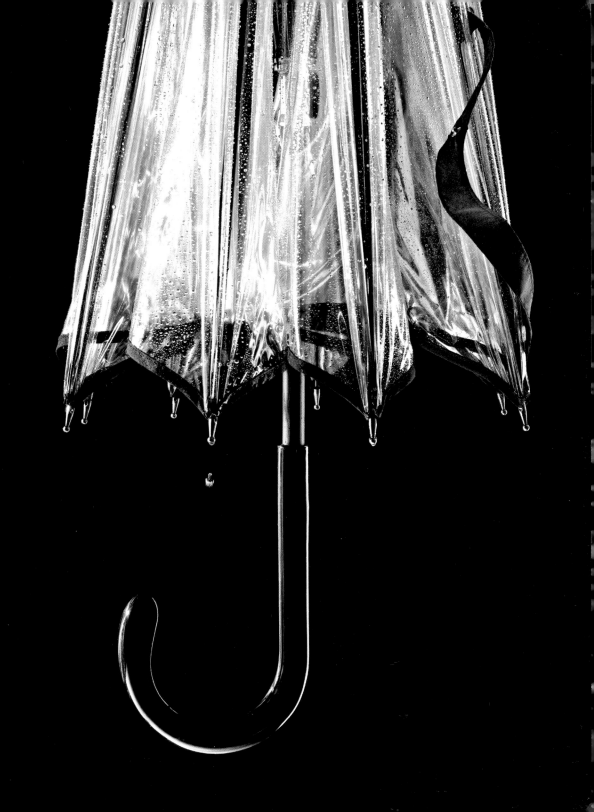

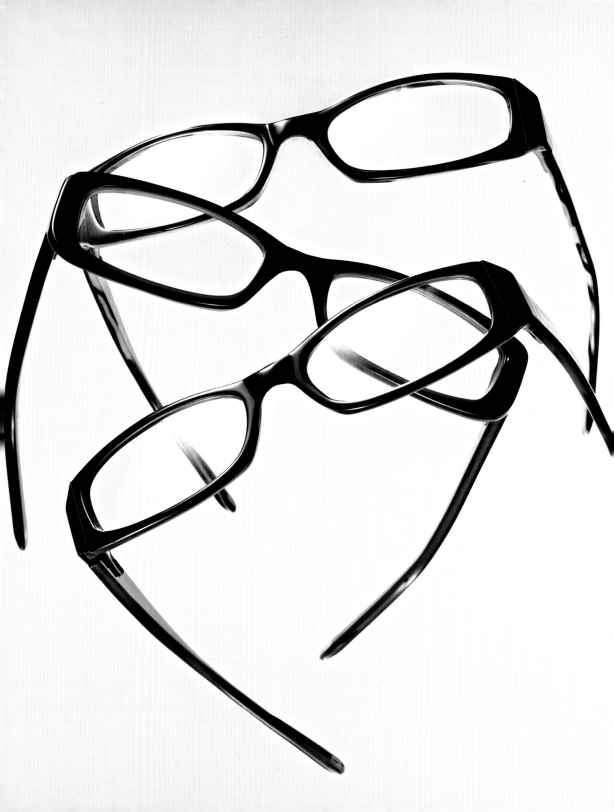

These aren't the singular pair of glasses that are handed to you before getting on the school bus that you must guard with your life. Your choice today might be the focal point of closing the next big deal, which could be in a conference room or by candlelight.

THE EYE-CATCHING EYEWEAR

GROUND RULES FOR EYEWEAR SHOPPING

- Bring something to allow yourself to put your hair up or back.

- Wear a top that is neutral and body skimming. Something as simple as a white or black T-shirt that fits to the figure will allow the frames to stand alone.

- Light, natural makeup should be the look of the day. There is nothing flattering about *any* eyewear atop the bare face you woke up with—unless you are sixteen and that is the face you honestly give to the world each day.

- When trying on frames, be sure to look at yourself in a full-length mirror to see how the frames play into your complete look, not just from your chin up. Glasses are accessories too. The scale, color, and shape will impact your other regular accessory choices from the nose down.

- Go bold! Frames in an intense color will warm a pale face.

- Darker frames with subtle back color add a hint of style to more traditional work settings.

- Tortoise and mottled surfaces bring soft texture to the face.

- Thicker plastic frames in color are acceptable for even the most conservative lady.

Perfect Partners

page 158

page 17

page 34

page 171

page 214

Nearly every item of clothing listed in this book can benefit from and be visually boosted by the help of one single professional; a tailor.

An expert tailor can sometimes look at the exact same garment that you think fits and see nuanced ways in which it actually doesn't—from casual khaki pants to the most elaborate

THE TAILORING

evening attire. Allow them to do this, and watch your style soar in ways you could never imagine, for accurately tailored clothing can look more expensive, trim the figure to appear slimmer, and conceal anxiety areas that chip away at your self-confidence on important days.

If you have never visited a professional tailor, you are not alone. Many are based within your favorite department stores, but this style expert feels that the best of the bunch are usually in small shops on older, small-town Main Streets or tucked away on "the other side of the tracks," carrying on a family tradition of tailoring passed down through generations before them.

When your style GPS finally helps you find your tailor of choice, here three easy things to remember before you get started.

MAKE YOUR TAILOR YOUR BFF (BEST FRIEND IN FIT) Don't be shy with your tailor; they are on *your* side. Tell them all your insecurities, and they will help you work around them. Like a medical doctor's office, this is a space to feel safe and honest about what you'd like to show off—and what you'd rather have fade away.

HACK AWAY YOUR GIVEAWAYS If you find a classic item in your closet that is headed to the donation bin, move it into the tailor bin and prepare to hack away. For instance, turn a boxy, dated suit jacket into a three-quarter-sleeve cropped swing jacket with vintage buttons. Make an ankle-length skirt into an age-appropriate mini, to be worn with tights and boots in cooler months. If you are ready to donate or ditch it anyway, have fun with your tailor and hack away while letting your inner fashion designer shine through.

DREAMS ARE FREE Allow your tailor to dream for you, like a great hairstylist, and advise you on what potential is hidden behind the seams. It could be anything from a more flattering fit to a more versatile garment that brings you more outfit possibilities. Just bring in your clothes raw and let the tailor inspire a new life for them. The cost of tailoring is lower than that of buying something new, so why not? If their ideas aren't to your liking, you haven't spent a penny.

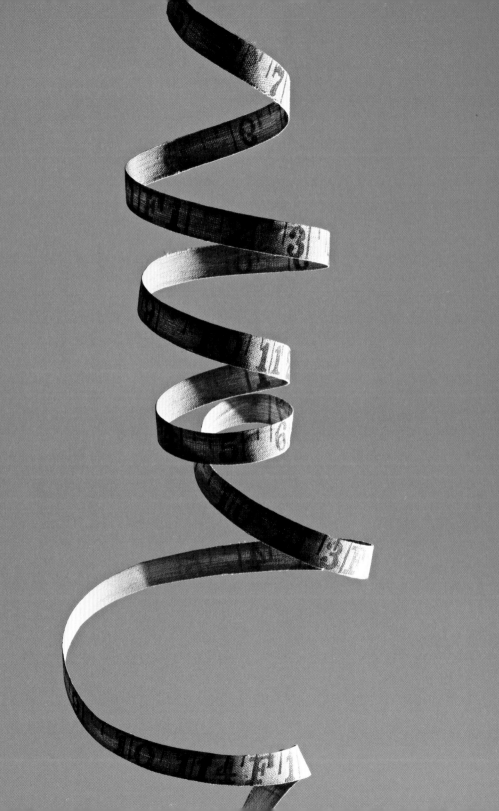

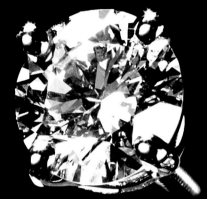

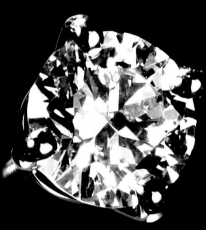

Perfect Partners

page 47   page 179   page 188   page 217   page 202

Let's make this one very simple. Tiffany diamond studs are a great investment to splurge on. There are only a few closet classics that must be called out by brand name. This is one of them, and for good reason. Most women who understand fine jewelry know that since 1837, Tiffany and Co. has been one of the world's most instantly recognizable and respected luxury brands. The world knows their logo, box color, and signature designs from miles away.

A well-turned-out closet can really be just one of each of the classics. One great white shirt, a single pair of amazing black stilettos, a singularly phenomenal straw

THE TIFFANY DIAMOND STUDS

bag for summer, and the list goes on. Style icons such as this don't need to be duplicated and owned in varied colors or fabrics. When you have the right one, you are finished, and investing in additional versions is really a matter of excessive fun.

If you own only these classic earrings, you honestly won't ever need another pair of any kind. Tiffany & Co. boasts that they are meticulously matched for size, color, clarity, and presence. The versions that speak the loudest to this style expert are usually set in platinum and made for pierced ears. Choosing round or square is a matter of personal preference.

A man who owns a perfectly tailored, year-round-weight, navy blue business suit and can't yet afford to purchase a suit in another color—he's fine. The Tiffany diamond studs are like your navy blue suit! These earrings make just as much sense when you put them on with your Bermuda shorts and striped T-shirt for a summer barbecue as they do when you slide them in at the last moment when getting dressed for a formal wedding, whether your own or that of a good gal pal.

Yes, you can keep a jewelry box of dangling bauble earrings, exotic chandelier drops, huggies, and even oversize hoops—they will always add fun winks to your look of the day. But if you decide to strip your clothing and accessory storehouse down to a stealth, focused collection of singularly timeless tools, you now know the only earring that you might ever need.

And here's a little secret: Just like the classic Billie Holiday song "Until the Real Thing Comes Along" says, investing in a more affordable, costume impostor is not a total no-no. For let's be real here. Just do your homework to make sure that they look as close to the genuine article as possible until the real thing is *comfortably* within your grasp.

Finish is about nuance. Envision the perfect hoop earring worn without a complementary watch, necklace, and anklet—simple. Or just a mist of a beautifully entrancing scent that barely dances from your body into the formerly blank airspace around you.

For one woman, this scent may be an extension of her just-showered aroma, a subtly soapy top note infused with hints of lavender, fresh cut grass, and jasmine. Whereas the next woman feels even sexier when she's caught in the first breath of a summer

THE SIGNATURE SCENT

rain, the smell you can detect before a drop even hits the ground. These moments speak of universal warmth for both the wearer and those who will involuntarily experience the scent.

Consider the world around you when choosing a signature scent, a faint sensory alert that will act as your fail-safe for the majority of your week. Remember, you may shift into something stronger or spicier for hot nights out, or opt for a sweeter, more floral moment when you are heading off on vacation, but your signature scent is your everyday common denominator, a stamp that becomes as constant as your handwriting, laugh, or smile. It may alter a bit from year to year, but those who know you could tell it from a mile away—in a good way.

Your clothing and accessories yearn for a polished finish—and this never means a load of last-minute touches. Just whispers of elegance that become what you are known for. Select yours in the privacy of your home by gathering samples on your next few shopping days, not at a crowded makeup counter in a bustling department store.

Try a new one for each of seven days straight, and use a mild, fragrance-free soap and moisturizer to welcome the full body and varied notes of its intended scent message.

Count the feedback and compliments, and let that influence your decision. If people ask, "What are you wearing?" you usually have struck a pleasing chord, for a day's worth of silence might be telling you the exact opposite. Err on the side of less rather than more, and always remember that you smell it less than those around you. Choose wisely.

Perfect Partners

page 33 page 117 page 41 page 3 page 205

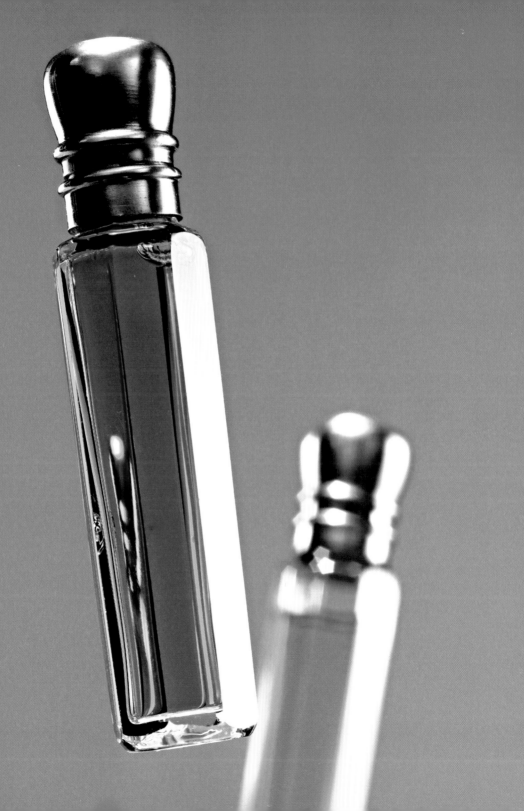

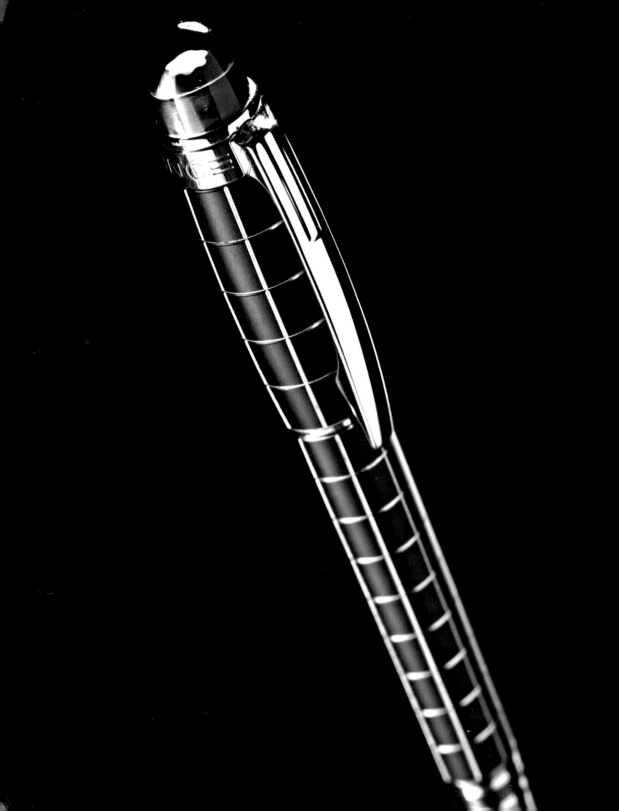

umbling and searching for a pen might be one of the most common activities that women perform, especially when chic, jumbo designer handbags are de rigueur. The pen you are searching for is usually buried deep beneath everything that you *don't* need at that moment, and the electronic device you *could* punch information into seems like more of a hassle in that moment than a time saver. When you finally do unearth the pen, which hopefully hasn't exploded

THE WRITING PEN

onto the bag itself, are you proud of it? If you aren't, was it worth all that time and frustration and possible cost to clean (or worse yet, replace) your satchel? It is beyond time to be proud of your plume! And trust that if you take the time to invest in a quality version, you will probably keep it housed in a slim felt bag or clamshell carrying case—so you not only get your time back and protect your bag, but also gain a few compliments in the process. Feel free to write me a lovely thank-you note.

Perfect Partners

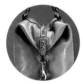

page 201   page 10   page 202   page 77   page 210

CHECKLIST

Use the following chart to check off items you have in your wardrobe.

1 WORK

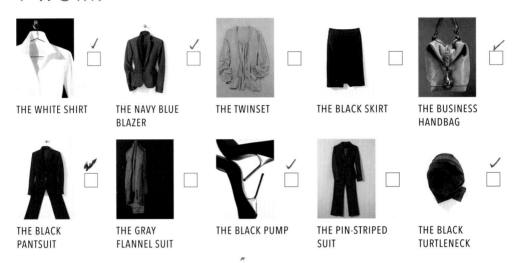

THE WHITE SHIRT

THE NAVY BLUE BLAZER

THE TWINSET

THE BLACK SKIRT

THE BUSINESS HANDBAG

THE BLACK PANTSUIT

THE GRAY FLANNEL SUIT

THE BLACK PUMP

THE PIN-STRIPED SUIT

THE BLACK TURTLENECK

2 WEEKEND

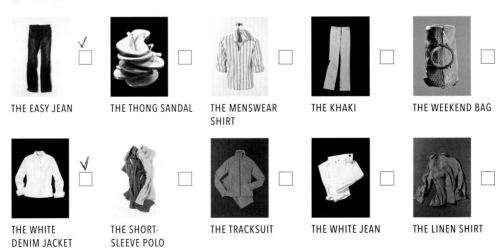

THE EASY JEAN

THE THONG SANDAL

THE MENSWEAR SHIRT

THE KHAKI

THE WEEKEND BAG

THE WHITE DENIM JACKET

THE SHORT-SLEEVE POLO

THE TRACKSUIT

THE WHITE JEAN

THE LINEN SHIRT

3 SATURDAY NIGHT

 ☐ THE PARTY DRESS

 ☐ THE SENSIBLY CHIC HEELS

 ☑ THE LEATHER JACKET

 ☑ THE SEQUINED TANK

 ☐ THE SCARF BLOUSE

 ☑ THE TRAFFIC-STOPPING JEAN

 ☑ THE CAMISOLE

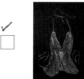 ☐ THE HALTER TOP

 ☐ THE JAW-DROPPING DRESS

 ☐ THE WIDE BELT

4 TRAVEL

 ☐ THE SAFARI JACKET

 ☑ THE TROUSER JEAN

 ☑ THE NUDE HEEL

 ☐ THE FABULOUS BEACH TOTE

 ☐ THE LONG LIGHTWEIGHT SCARF

 ☐ THE FESTIVE FLAT

 ☑ THE SHAWL WRAP SWEATER

 ☐ THE BOLD TRENCH

 ☐ THE DRIVING MOCCASIN

 ☑ THE MODERN BEACH COVER-UP

5 PUNCTUATION

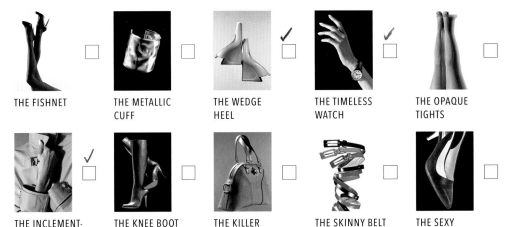

THE FISHNET   THE METALLIC CUFF   THE WEDGE HEEL ✓   THE TIMELESS WATCH ✓   THE OPAQUE TIGHTS

THE INCLEMENT-WEATHER ENTRANCE-MAKER ✓   THE KNEE BOOT   THE KILLER WORK TOTE   THE SKINNY BELT   THE SEXY SLINGBACK

6 ACTIVE (OR NOT)

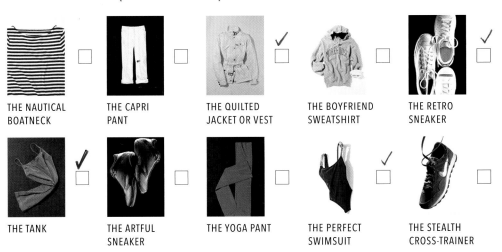

THE NAUTICAL BOATNECK   THE CAPRI PANT   THE QUILTED JACKET OR VEST ✓   THE BOYFRIEND SWEATSHIRT   THE RETRO SNEAKER ✓

THE TANK ✓   THE ARTFUL SNEAKER   THE YOGA PANT   THE PERFECT SWIMSUIT ✓   THE STEALTH CROSS-TRAINER

7 ENTERTAINING

 ☐ THE DRESSY
FLAT SANDAL

 ☐ THE RUFFLED TOP

 ☐ THE FLORAL
STATEMENT PIECE

 ✓ THE ESPADRILLE

 ☐ THE FAIL-SAFE
HURRIED-HOSTESS TOP

 ☐ THE MUST-HAVE
MULE

 ☐ THE LINEN PANT

 ✓ THE BERMUDA
SHORT

 ☐ THE "GROWN-UP"
PAJAMA

 ☐ THE "FROCK"
TUNIC DRESS

8 POWER MOVES

 ☐ MODERN PEARLS

 ✓ THE WRAP DRESS

 ✓ THE COCKTAIL RING

 ✓ THE ANIMAL PRINT

 ☐ THE MENSWEAR PANT

 ☐ THE EPIC
CHANDELIER
EARRING

 ✓ THE CHANEL JACKET

 ☐ THE POWER OF RED

 ☐ THE CAMEL COAT

 ☐ THE VINTAGE
CONVERSATION PIECE

9 EVENING

 ✓
☐

THE METALLIC
EVENING SHOE

 ✓
☐

THE EVENING SHOE

☐

THE CREAM
DRESS PANT

☐

THE EVENING
GOWN

 ✓
☐

THE BLACK
VELVET BLAZER

 ✓
☐

THE STATEMENT
EVENING BAG

☐

THE *MODERN*
EVENING WRAP

☐

THE BALL GOWN
SKIRT

☐

THE LADYLIKE
EVENING COAT

 ✓
☐

THE LITTLE
BLACK DRESS

10 THE FINISHING TOUCHES

☐

THE SOPHISTICATED
WALLET

☐

THE ENVY-INSPIRING
SUNGLASSES

☐

THE HOOP
EARRING

☐

THE TRIO OF
WOODEN BANGLES

☐

THE PERFECT
UMBRELLA

☐

THE EYE-CATCHING
EYEWEAR

☐

THE TAILORING

☐

THE TIFFANY
DIAMOND STUDS

 ✓
☐

THE SIGNATURE
SCENT

☐

THE WRITING PEN

ACKNOWLEDGMENTS

Thank you, God! I wrote this book in N.Y., L.A., Key West, and (literally) while flying over nearly every state in between. You kept me safe and blessed—and I thank you.

To the smart and stylish team at Atria Books: Judith Curr, Malaika Adero (my editor par excellence), Christine Lloreda, Jeanne Lee, Lisa Sciambra, Rachel Bostic, and Todd Hunter. Many thanks for giving me another platform to share my style philosophy with readers everywhere.

Faith Childs, you are the best literary agent an author could dream of. This is our fourth book—and the best yet—thanks to all of your hard work and vision. Check!

Robert Tardio, your masterful eye, meticulous attention to detail, and breathtaking photography brought this book to life. Let's not wait another ten years to create magic! Thanks also to your incredible assistant, Tiffany Latz, a whirlwind of energy and organization—with a smile all the while. To your sharp still-life stylists, Renata Chaplynsky and Megan Krieman—you ladies are incredible at what you do: thanks so very much for adding the polish to my dream. And a huge thanks to your agent, the chic Janice Moses, for keeping it all together.

Sharon Pendana, the stylist's stylist! Your "magic" is legendary. Your eye remains extraordinary. We have always made a great team, and this book is our best work yet. More to come, Pen-Chattie!

Thanks to my family at Jones New York: Stacy Lastrina, Amy Rapawy, Susan Metzger, Shirley Imig, Jolene Zupnik, and Stephanie McInerny. Thank you for choosing and trusting me to represent your brand from coast to coast for all these years, and for taking such good care of me every step of the way. You helped to bring this book to life, so it is ours to celebrate! *Let's go shopping!*

To my ever-chic mom, Lynell Boston-Kollar, and the entire Mason-Johnson clan, here's the fourth book for your coffee tables. We did it again! Mom, thanks for loving me all the way through the stressful months wrapping this project. And for letting me simply be *me* from day one.

Jonathan, my partner, my cocktail maker, and my true love—thanks for rubbing my feet when the stress simply got to be too much. And Kim Robson: Who knew I'd get a bonus, stylish sister out of the deal too! Thank you both.

Jackie Connolly, my secret-agent assistant. You worked like a cyber thief in the night on this book, getting everything done with calm and focus. Thanks for sticking with me!

To my über-incredible TV agent, Katie Maloney: You are really the best at what you do. Honored to be with you. Thanks also to Lia "Boots" Aponte, and my team at NS Bienstock. Thanks for keeping me hosting quality TV!

Jeff Googel, my main man and commercial/endorsement agent at William Morris Endeavor Entertainment, thanks for having my back at every turn for all these years—you are incredible. Thanks also to Jeff Lesh at WMEE for keeping me booked on fun, stylish speaking gigs, style seminars, and book signings!

Tommy Hilfiger, my former boss of more than a decade and forever mentor and friend. Wouldn't be here without you. Thanks for always keeping one eye on my brand too! Love ya, T. H.!

Cynde Watson and Craig Rose, my siblings to the end—you are both next as authors. Can't wait to throw *your* book events! And my posse of supportive chosen family: Steve Barr, Ludlow Beckett, Nicole Blades, Gordon Chambers, Rodney Chester, Allen Harvey, Bobby Johnson, Doug Jones, Darryl Parker, Patrick-Ian Polk, Troy Powell, Urbano Steriti, and Russ Torres. Thanks so very much! If I forgot you, please just blame it on the burnout.

Thanks to all designers, stores, and brands that generously lent their classics to me—I hope the beautiful photography and credit listing is worth a thousand thanks! To my models, Viki and Sherrylene—you brought the sizzle, thanks!

Lastly, but never least, to my loyal readers, lloydboston.com visitors, and TV viewers, I so appreciate you trusting *me* to guide you. In a sea of experts, you have chosen to stick with me for over a decade. Know that I will never let you leave the house without a confident, stylish finish. Stay close!

STYLE SOURCES

Apsan, Rebecca. *The Lingerie Handbook.* New York: Workman, 2006.

Calasibetta, Charlotte Mankey. *Fairchild's Dictionary of Fashion.* New York: Fairchild Books, 2000.

Chierichetti, David. *Edith Head: The Life and Times of Hollywood's Celebrated Costume Designer.* New York: HarperCollins, 2003.

"Coco Chanel Quotes." Thinkexist.com. thinkexist.com/quotes/coco_chanel/.

Corrigan, Joyce. "Golden Time at the Studio Museum." Artnet.com. www.artnet.com/magazine/features/corrigan/corrigan4-12-00.asp.

Garland, Phyl. "Is the Afro on the Way Out?" *Ebony*, February 1973: 128–36.

Glasses. New York: Stewart, Tabori & Chang, 1999.

Head, Edith. *The Dress Doctor.* New York: Collins Design, 2008.

"History of Earrings." *Diamond Earrings* blog, July 22, 2005. professorices.blogspot.com/2005/07/history-of-earrings.html.

"History of Earrings." Surfindia.com. www.surfindia.com/matrimonials/history-of-earrings.html.

Kirschner, Marilyn. "*WWD: The Magazine* . . . Worth the 10 Bucks?" Lookonline.com. www.lookonline.com/wwd.html.

Larocca, Amy. "68 Minutes with Anna Wintour." *New York*, September 14, 2009: 24.

Loughran, Maire. "Cuff Bracelets: Jewelry from the Balenciaga Fall Fashion Show." Suite101.com, May 28, 2009. bracelets.suite101.com/article.cfm/cuff_bracelets.

"Marlene Dietrich Quotes." Quoteopia.com. www.quoteopia.com/famous.php?quotesby=marlenedietrich.

Martin, Richard. "Vionnet, Madeleine." From *Contemporary Fashion* (2002), quoted on Encyclopedia.com. www.encyclopedia.com/doc/1G2-3401400437.html.

McDonald, Brian. "Umbrella Repair Tips: Fix Your Favorite Rain Umbrella." www.howtodothings.com/family-and-relationships/a4487-how-to-repair-an-umbrella.html.

Miller, Amanda Christine. "Diane von Furstenberg On Wrap Dresses And The Joys Of Aging Gracefully." *Huffington Post*, January 16, 2008. www.huffingtonpost.com/amanda-christine-miller/diane-von-furstenberg-on-_b_81590.html.

Moe, Jack. "Cross Training Shoes." Speedysneakers.com, November 14, 2009. www.speedysneakers.com/ArticlesForum/tabid/158/ctl/ReadDefault/mid/741/ArticleId/3/Default.aspx.

Muller, Florence. *Fashion Game Book: A World History of Twentieth-Century Fashion*. New York: Assouline, 2008.

"Navy Uniform History." About.com. usmilitary.about.com/od/navy/l/bluniformhist.htm.

Nelson, Karin. "The World Is Flat." *New York Times*, August 9, 2009, New Jersey edition, sec. 3.

Palileo, Bettina. "What Length Are Capri Pants?" EHow.com. www.ehow.com/about_5214770_length-capri-pants_.html.

"Quotes About 'Dress.'" Quoteopia.com. www.quoteopia.com/quotations.php?type=q&query=dress.

Robson, Julia. "A New Wave of Seaside Chic." Telegraph.co.uk, June 11, 2004. www.telegraph.co.uk/fashion/3325705/A-new-wave-of-seaside-chic.html.

Rosenbloom, Stephanie. "Tightening Belts? She's the Expert." *New York Times*, July 18, 2009, New Jersey edition, sec. 1.

Shoes. New York: Stewart, Tabori & Chang, 1999.

"Tiffany Solitaire Diamond Earrings." Tiffany.com. www.tiffany.com/Shopping/Item.aspx?fromGrid=1&sku=GRP00432&mcat=148210&cid=287464&search_params=s+2-p+4-c+-r+101287464+10132 3351-x+-n+6-ri+-ni+0-t+.

"What Michelle Obama's Wearing Now." *Flypaper* blog, March 31, 2009. flypaper.bluefly.com/archives/2009/03/what-michelle-obama-is-wearing-now.html.

"Women's Pajamas: A Multi-Billion-Dollar Industry." Press release, July 9, 2009. www.free-press-release.com/news/200512/1134571005.html.

"Yoga Info 101." Lululemon.com. www.lululemon.com/education/yoga.

DESIGNER LISTING

PHOTOGRAPHY CREDITS

All Original Photography for Cover and Interior

Robert Tardio

All Makeup and Grooming for Author and Models

Cynde Watson/cyndewatson.com

Archival Photography

Page xviii: © 2000 Mark Shaw/mptvimages.com

Page 22: © 2000 Mark Shaw/mptvimages.com

Page 44: mptvimages.com

Page 66: © 1978 David Sutton/mptviamges.com

Page 88: Otto Dyar/Getty Images

Page 110: Chris Walter/Getty Images

Page 132: © 1978 John Engstead/mptviamges.com

Page 154: Pascal Le Segretain/Getty Images

Page 176: mptvimages.com

Page 198: A. L. Whitey Schafer/Getty Images

INDEX

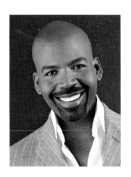

LLOYD BOSTON • AUTHOR

is a top TV style expert, television host, and the author of three popular style books—including *Before You Put That On*. The former vice president of art direction for Tommy Hilfiger, he's been a regular on-air style contributor for NBC's *Today* show with over 150 segments to his credit, and made several appearances on *Oprah*, *The View*, and CNN. An original host on the STYLE Network, Lloyd has also been the host of his own show, *Closet Cases*, and several specials for the Fine Living Network and HGTV. He is currently the red carpet commentator for NBCs *Extra* and the exclusive Style Guy for Jones New York, helping women to craft their style. Lloyd splits his time between New York and Los Angeles.

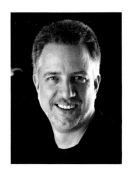

ROBERT TARDIO • PHOTOGRAPHER

Photographer Robert Tardio was raised in the outskirts of Washington, DC. He attended Colgate University where he studied art history, photography, and film, and received his B.A. with Honors in Fine Arts. Robert moved to New York City to pursue work as a photographer and opened his New York studio in 1987. He works on advertising, editorial, and design assignments and has received numerous awards in recognition of his creative efforts including a Clio and an MPA Kelly Award. He has also been recognized by numerous publications, including *Print* magazine, *Communication Arts*, *Art Direction*, *Graphis*, PDN/Nikon, and the APA awards book.

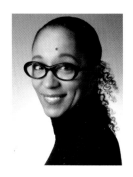

SHARON PENDANA • STYLE EDITOR

Sharon Pendana is a seasoned fashion professional bringing years of sartorial expertise to her work as a wardrobe stylist and costume designer (USA Local 829) for print, film, and television. She is a partner in Full Circle Six, a consortium of lifestyle professionals and is a frequent collaborator with Lloyd Boston.